Chronic Myelogenous Leukemia

Guest Editor

DANIEL J. DEANGELO, MD, PhD

HEMATOLOGY/ONCOLOGY CLINICS OF NORTH AMERICA

www.hemonc.theclinics.com

Consulting Editors
GEORGE P. CANELLOS, MD
NANCY BERLINER, MD

October 2011 • Volume 25 • Number 5

SAUNDERS an imprint of ELSEVIER, Inc.

W.B. SAUNDERS COMPANY
A Division of Elsevier Inc.

1600 John F. Kennedy Blvd. • Suite 1800 • Philadelphia, PA 19103-2899

http://www.theclinics.com

HEMATOLOGY/ONCOLOGY CLINICS OF NORTH AMERICA Volume 25, Number 5
October 2011 ISSN 0889-8588, ISBN 13: 978-1-4377-2530-8

Editor: Patrick Manley

Hematology/Oncology Clinics (ISSN 0889-8588) is published bimonthly by Elsevier Inc., 360 Park Avenue South, New York, NY 10010-1710. Months of issue are February, April, June, August, October, and December. Business and Editorial Offices: 1600 John F. Kennedy Blvd., Ste. 1800, Philadelphia, PA 19103—2899. Customer Service Office: 3251 Riverport Lane, Maryland Heights, MO 63043. Periodicals postage paid at New York, NY and at additional mailing offices. Subscription prices are $327.00 per year (domestic individuals), $541.00 per year (domestic institutions), $160.00 per year (domestic students/residents), $371.00 per year (Canadian individuals), $662.00 per year (Canadian institutions) $442.00 per year (international individuals), $662.00 per year (international institutions), and $216.00 per year (international and Canadian students/residents). International air speed delivery is included in all *Clinics* subscription prices. All prices are subject to change without notice. **POSTMASTER:** Send address changes to *Hematology/Oncology Clinics of North America*, Elsevier Health Sciences Division, Subscription Customer Service, 3251 Riverport Lane, Maryland Heights, MO 63043. Customer Service (orders, claims, online, change of address): Elsevier Health Sciences Division, Subscription Customer Service, 3251 Riverport Lane, Maryland Heights, MO 63043. Tel: 1-800-654-2452 (U.S. and Canada); 314-447-8871 (outside U.S. and Canada). Fax: 314-447-8029. E-mail: journalscustomerservice-usa@elsevier.com (for print support); journalsonlinesupport-usa@elsevier.com (for online support).

Reprints. For copies of 100 or more, of articles in this publication, please contact the Commercial Reprints Department, Elsevier Inc., 360 Park Avenue South, New York, New York 10010-1710; Tel.: 212-633-3813, Fax: 212-462-1935, E-mail: reprints@elsevier.com.

Hematology/Oncology Clinics of North America is covered in *MEDLINE/PubMed (Index Medicus), EMBASE/ Excerpta Medica, and BIOSIS.*

Printed and bound by CPI Group (UK) Ltd, Croydon, CR0 4YY

Transferred to Digital Print 2011

Contributors

CONSULTING EDITORS

GEORGE P. CANELLOS, MD
William Rosenberg Professor of Medicine, Department of Medical Oncology, Dana-Farber Cancer Institute, Boston, Massachusetts

NANCY BERLINER, MD
Chief, Division of Hematology, Brigham and Women's Hospital; Professor of Medicine, Harvard Medical School, Boston, Massachusetts

GUEST EDITOR

DANIEL J. DEANGELO, MD, PhD
Associate Professor of Medicine, Harvard Medical School; Clinical Director, Adult Leukemia Program, Dana-Farber Cancer Institute, Brigham and Women's Hospital, Boston, Massachusetts

AUTHORS

SHEELA A. ABRAHAM, PhD
Section of Experimental Haematology, Cancer Division, Faculty of Medicine, University of Glasgow, Paul O'Gorman Leukaemia Research Centre, Gartnavel General Hospital, Glasgow; Stem Cell and Leukaemia Proteomics Laboratory, School of Cancer and Enabling Sciences, Manchester Academic Health Science Centre, The University of Manchester, Christie's NHS Foundation Trust, Wolfson Molecular Imaging Centre, Withington, Manchester, United Kingdom

PAULO LISBOA BITTENCOURT, MD, PhD
Unit of Gastroenterology and Hepatology, Portuguese Hospital, Salvador, Bahia, Brazil

JORGE CORTES, MD
The University of Texas MD Anderson Cancer Center, Houston, Texas

CLÁUDIA ALVES COUTO, MD, PhD
Alfa Gastroenterology Institute, Federal University of Minas Gerais, Belo Horizonte, Minas Gerais, Brazil

MICHAEL W.N. DEININGER, MD, PhD
M.M Wintrobe Professor of Medicine, Chief, Division of Hematology and Hematologic Malignancies, Huntsman Cancer Institute, University of Utah, Salt Lake City, Utah

THOMAS ERNST, Dr. med
Klinik für Innere Medizin II, Universitätsklinikum Jena, Jena, Germany

PAOLO GALLIPOLI, MD
Section of Experimental Haematology, Cancer Division, Faculty of Medicine, University of Glasgow, Paul O'Gorman Leukaemia Research Centre, Gartnavel General Hospital, Glasgow, United Kingdom

TRACY I. GEORGE, MD
Assistant Professor, Department of Pathology, Stanford University School of Medicine, Stanford University Medical Center, Stanford, California

ANDREAS HOCHHAUS, Dr. med
Klinik für Innere Medizin II, Universitätsklinikum Jena, Jena, Germany

TESSA L. HOLYOAKE, PhD, MD
Section of Experimental Haematology, Cancer Division, Faculty of Medicine, University of Glasgow, Paul O'Gorman Leukaemia Research Centre, Gartnavel General Hospital, Glasgow, United Kingdom

HANS-PETER HORNY, MD
Professor, Institut für Pathologie, Klinikum Ansbach, Escherichstrasse, Ansbach, Germany

ELIAS JABBOUR, MD
The University of Texas MD Anderson Cancer Center, Houston, Texas

NITIN JAIN, MD
Section of Hematology/Oncology, University of Chicago, Chicago, Illinois

HAGOP KANTARJIAN, MD
The University of Texas MD Anderson Cancer Center, Houston, Texas

JAMSHID S. KHORASHAD, MD, PhD
Post Doctoral Research Fellow, Deininger Lab, Huntsman Cancer Institute, University of Utah, Salt Lake City, Utah

PAUL LA ROSÉE, Dr. med
Klinik für Innere Medizin II, Universitätsklinikum Jena, Jena, Germany

MARTIN C. MÜLLER, Dr. med
III Medizinische Klinik, Universitätsmedizin Mannheim, Mannheim, Germany

SAMEER A. PARIKH, MD
The University of Texas MD Anderson Cancer Center, Houston, Texas

JERALD P. RADICH, MD
Clinical Research Division, Fred Hutchinson Cancer Research Center, Seattle, Washington

DANIEL DIAS RIBEIRO, MD, PhD
Alfa Gastroenterology Institute; Department of Hematology, Federal University of Minas Gerais, Belo Horizonte, Minas Gerais, Brazil

KOEN VAN BESIEN, MD
Section of Hematology/Oncology, University of Chicago, Chicago, Illinois

SA A. WANG, MD
Associate Director of Clinical Flow Cytometry Laboratory, Department of Hematopathology, University of Texas MD Anderson Cancer Center, Houston, Texas

Contents

refractory to imatinib or eventually relapse. Resistance is frequently associated with mutations in the kinase domain of BCR-ABL. Over 100 point mutations coding for single amino acid substitutions in the BCR-ABL kinase domain have been isolated from CML patients resistant to imatinib treatment. Most reported mutants are rare, whereas 7 mutated residues comprise two-thirds of all mutations detected. BCR-ABL mutations affect amino acids involved in imatinib binding or in regulatory regions of the BCR-ABL kinase domain, resulting in decreased sensitivity to imatinib while retaining aberrant kinase activity. The early detection of BCR-ABL mutants during therapy may aid in risk stratification as well as molecularly based treatment decisions.

This article reviews to what extent molecular data can be used to rationalize therapeutic choices in the treatment of chronic myeloid leukemia. Two categories of data are discussed: markers that globally measure risk but do not provide a molecular rationale for therapy selection; and biomarkers with a causal link to a clinical phenotype, such as certain mutations of the BCR-ABL kinase domain. As therapy selection is still mainly based on clinical criteria, molecular biomarkers are discussed in the context of available clinical prognostication tools, focusing on biomarkers that do not reflect disease burden as a surrogate of responsiveness to treatment.

In the pre-tyrosine kinase (TKI) era, allogeneic stem cell transplant (allo-SCT) was the front-line treatment of choice for young patients with chronic myelogenous leukemia (CML). Today, imatinib is well established as front-line therapy for CML, with excellent long-term outcomes. This has changed the role of allo-SCT and the number of patients undergoing allo-SCT has declined dramatically. Allo-SCT is currently recommended for patients in accelerated/blast phase disease, those who have failed a second-generation TKI and those with TKI-resistant mutations such as T315I. The role of allo-SCT in the management of CML will require continual reappraisal as medical therapies continue to evolve.

Venous thrombosis results from the convergence of vessel wall injury and/or venous stasis, known as local triggering factors, and the occurrence of acquired and/or inherited thrombophilia, also known as systemic prothrombotic risk factors. Portal vein thrombosis (PVT) and Budd–Chiari syndrome (BCS) are caused by thrombosis and/or obstruction of the extrahepatic portal veins and the hepatic venous outflow tract, respectively. Several divergent prothrombotic disorders may underlie these distinct forms of large vessel thrombosis. While cirrhotic PVT is relatively common, especially in advanced liver disease, noncirrhotic and nontumoral PVT is rare and BCS is of intermediate incidence. In this article, we review pathogenic mechanisms and current concepts of patient management.

An unusual disease, mastocytosis challenges the pathologist with a variety of morphologic appearances and heterogeneous clinical presentations ranging from skin manifestations (pruritus, urticaria, dermatographism) to systemic signs and symptoms indicative of mast cell mediator release, including flushing, hypotension, headache, and anaphylaxis among others. In this article, we focus on recognizing the cytology, histopathology, clinical features, and prognostic implications of systemic mastocytosis, a clonal and neoplastic mast cell proliferation infiltrating extracutaneous organ(s) with or without skin involvement. Diagnostic pitfalls are reviewed with ancillary studies to help unmask the mast cell and exclude morphologic mimics.

Sustained clinical cytopenia is a frequent laboratory finding in ambulatory and hospitalized patients. For pathologists and hematopathologists who examine the bone marrow (BM), a diagnosis of cytopenia secondary to an infiltrative BM process or acute leukemia can be readily established based on morphologic evaluation and flow cytometry immunophenotyping. However, it can be more challenging to establish a diagnosis of myelodysplastic syndrome (MDS). In this article, the practical approaches for establishing or excluding a diagnosis of MDS (especially low-grade MDS) in patients with clinical cytopenia are discussed along with the current diagnostic recommendations provided by the World Health Organization and the International Working Group for MDS.

THE CLINICS ARE NOW AVAILABLE ONLINE!

Access your subscription at:
www.theclinics.com

Preface

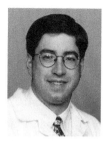

Daniel J. DeAngelo, MD, PhD
Guest Editor

The development of imatinib mesylate (Gleevac, STI571) for the treatment of patients with Philadelphia-positive chronic myelogenous leukemia (CML) introduced a paradigm shift in medical oncology. For the first time, we had an oral agent that was not only well tolerated, but incredibly efficacious. Imatinib mesylate is a selective BCR-ABL inhibitor that results in a 98% complete hematologic remission and, more importantly, an 87% complete cytogenetic remission rate. The results with imatinib mesylate have been so extraordinary that allogeneic stem cell transplant, historically the recommended upfront strategy, is now only used in refractory cases. In addition to the Abl kinase, imatinib inhibits the tyrosine kinase activity of many other diseases, including gastrointestinal stromal cell tumors, myeloproliferative disorders including chronic myelomonocytic leukemia that contains a PDGFRB gene rearrangement, hypereosinophilic syndrome, and mast cell disorders.

Unfortunately, even though an increasing portion of patients with CML is able to achieve a cytogenetic and molecular remission, imatinib mesylate therapy remains a life-long endeavor. Few patients are actually "cured" with this approach, as the quiescent leukemia stem cell seems unaffected by tyrosine kinase inhibition. Nevertheless, CML is becoming a chronic disease with an ever-increasing disease prevalence. Approximately 95% of patients with CML are alive and well more than 5 years from their initial disease diagnosis, which is a dramatic improvement from the median 3- to 5-year survival only a decade ago.

In this issue of *Hematology/Oncology Clinics of North America*, concepts regarding the pathophysiology of resistance, therapeutic approaches, and future investigational therapies are discussed. Experts in the field of CML research were invited to share their views on a wide range of selected topics. In addition, the topics on mastocytosis and

Hematol Oncol Clin N Am 25 (2011) ix–x
doi:10.1016/j.hoc.2011.10.001
0889-8588/11/$ – see front matter
hemonc.theclinics.com

portal vein thrombosis have also been included, which round out this edition. I hope that you will find these reviews constructive as well as enjoyable.

With regards,

Daniel J. DeAngelo, MD, PhD
Adult Leukemia Program
Dana-Farber Cancer Institute
Brigham and Women's Hospital
450 Brookline Avenue
Boston, MA 02115-5450, USA

E-mail address:
Daniel_Deangelo@dfci.harvard.edu

Hurdles Toward a Cure for CML: The CML Stem Cell

Paolo Gallipoli, MD[a], Sheela A. Abraham, PhD[a,b],
Tessa L. Holyoake, PhD, MD[a,*]

KEYWORDS

- Chronic myeloid leukemia • Stem cell • Targeted therapy
- Cure

Chronic myeloid leukemia (CML) is recognized as a disease model for oncogene addiction, targeted therapy, and cancer stem cells (CSCs). As the first cancer in which a genetic alteration was proven to be of pathogenic significance, CML research has remained at the leading edge, providing great insights into cellular and molecular biology and most recently in systems biology. CML, driven by genomic instability induced by the BCR-ABL oncogene, naturally progresses over time from chronic phase to accelerated phase (CP and AP) and eventually to blast crisis (BC).[1] Following many frustrating years in the 1970s and 1980s, during which we used toxic strategies, such as high-dose chemotherapy, allogeneic stem cell transplantation (alloSCT) and autologous transplantation, interferon-α (IFN-α), and cytosine arabinoside, the late 1990s saw the introduction of targeted therapies, the tyrosine kinase inhibitors (TKIs), including imatinib mesylate (IM) (Gleevec, Novartis, Basel, Switzerland), dasatinib (DAS) (Sprycel, Bristol-Myers Squibb, New York, NY, USA), and nilotinib (NIL) (Tasigna, Novartis, Basel, Switzerland). These agents have dramatically altered the natural history of CML in CP, such that many individuals now experience a near normal quality of life with very significantly improved overall survival (OS).[2] These agents are expensive, however, and therefore are not accessible to patients in many parts of the world. For patients fortunate enough to receive continuous treatment with TKIs, 30% to 60% experience grade 1–2 and 10% to 20% experience grade 3–4 side effects.[2] Drug adherence studies also demonstrate reduced compliance over time, such that by 5 years of

The authors have nothing to disclose.

[a] Section of Experimental Haematology, Cancer Division, Faculty of Medicine, University of Glasgow, Paul O'Gorman Leukaemia Research Centre, Gartnavel General Hospital, 1053 Great Western Road, Glasgow, G12 0YN, UK

[b] Stem Cell and Leukaemia Proteomics Laboratory, School of Cancer and Enabling Sciences, Manchester Academic Health Science Centre, The University of Manchester, Christie's NHS Foundation Trust, Wolfson Molecular Imaging Centre, 27 Palatine Road, Withington, Manchester, M20 3LJ, UK

* Corresponding author.
E-mail address: tlh1g@clinmed.gla.ac.uk

continuous therapy only 70% of patients are compliant and only 1 in 7 patients takes their medication exactly as instructed. In this situation, levels of compliance are very strongly correlated with disease response, suggesting that this is a critical issue for the ever-growing population of patients living with CML.[3,4]

CML arises in a hematopoietic stem cell (HSC) as a result of the 9;22 translocation. The resultant BCR-ABL tyrosine kinase drives myeloid expansion through to terminally differentiated cells, explaining the disease phenotype. The disease follows a near normal differentiation hierarchy, with mutant HSCs (often referred to as leukemic stem cells [LSCs]) sustaining and driving the disease.[5] This hierarchy is beautifully illustrated in patients on introduction of TKI therapy. In terms of leukemic burden, sensitively quantified by quantitative real-time polymerase chain reaction (Q-RT-PCR), there is a rapid decline explained by eradication of more mature BCR-ABL–positive cells, followed by a much slower reduction in CML progenitor cells to 3 years. Beyond 3 years, it is unclear whether the slope continues very slowly downward with cure predicted by 17 to 20 years, or whether disease levels plateau, presumably because CML LSCs represent a highly drug-refractory population.[6,7] What is very clear is that CML, even in CP, is a highly heterogeneous disease and this may well explain the variable disease kinetics observed in individual patients treated with TKIs and in the small proportion of patients with CML who have discontinued TKIs after several years of therapy.

In this article, we aim to review the relevant literature and define the role of CML LSCs as a hurdle to cure of this disease.

HISTORICAL PERSPECTIVE OF GENESIS AND HETEROGENEITY OF CANCER

Cancer is the result of perturbed cell growth processes. All tumors, whether solid or hematological, demonstrate substantial heterogeneity with respect to cell surface markers, morphology, genetic or epigenetic aberrations, cell growth kinetics, tumor-initiating capacity, and response to therapeutic agents.[8]

Past perspectives defining cancer and how it originates have laid the groundwork for contemporary models addressing tumor heterogeneity. In the early 19th century, Johannes Muller and Rudolf Virchow hypothesized that cancer arises from embryo-like cells, thereby initiating early concepts of CSC. In 1963, stem cell pioneers Becker and colleagues[9] described techniques involving a small population of normal hematopoietic cells that could form colonies in the spleen when injected into irradiated mice.[9] They determined that these cells had the ability to self-renew and differentiate into mature hematopoietic cells, thus establishing basic stem cell properties. In 1976, Peter Nowel hypothesized that cancer may change its capacity to grow and metastasize as the result of accumulated genetic mutations that produce a dominant tumor clone, through diversification and natural selection processes, fundamentally modeling carcinogenesis on Darwinian principles.[10] His landmark article suggested that tumor progression is based on neoplastic populations possessing an increased proliferative capacity and therefore exhibiting increased levels of fitness, leading to their selection. The universal acceptance that cancer is defined by abnormal growth control, resulted in therapies focused on augmented proliferation rates. Likewise, dosing and drug schedules were designed aiming for maximal tumor cell death with minimal toxicity to normal tissue.

Recently, a paradigm shift has occurred in the way cancer is perceived and how therapy might be redirected. This change in philosophy followed fundamental studies by Dick and colleagues demonstrating that acute myeloid leukemia (AML) contains a specialized population of cells expressing stem cell markers and exhibiting properties that can be propagated when transferred to immunocompromised NOD/SCID mice to cause leukemia.[11,12] This was the first formal demonstration that cancer cells within a tumor may follow a normal stem cell hierarchy.

CONTEMPORARY MODELS TO ACCOUNT FOR TUMOR HETEROGENEITY

Currently, 2 models that attempt to explain tumor heterogeneity dominate the field. The CSC model proposes that tumors follow a normal stem cell hierarchy, with CSCs having the sole ability to propagate themselves and reconstitute the entire tumor. In this model, CSCs are biologically distinct from the bulk tumor cells, can give rise to other CSCs through self-renewal, and can generate differentiated tumor cells. Proponents of this model emphasize that CSCs function as a distinct population, irrespective of their absolute frequency, with the primary tenets of the model being that the CSCs can be isolated, self-propagate, and initiate malignant growth.[13,14] More importantly, findings suggest that the presence of CSCs drives clinical cancer progression and contributes to treatment failure. It is important to emphasize that a CSC need not originate from a normal tissue stem cell that has undergone transformation, but may instead arise in a more mature cell that has re-acquired gene expression and functional characteristics that support self-renewal.[15] CSCs may arise from a stem cell, a committed progenitor, or even a terminally differentiated cell.[16] Cancers supporting the CSC model include leukemia; breast, ovarian, bladder, central nervous system, colon, head and neck, pancreatic, and liver cancer; and Ewing sarcoma.[17]

The clonal or stochastic model suggests that individual tumor cells are biologically equivalent, but subject to either intrinsic (transcription factors, regulatory pathways) or extrinsic factors (tumor milieu, immune response, microenvironment) that influence their fate. These indiscriminately induced, nonpermanent alterations to the cells eventually generate heterogeneity. In theory, every cell in the tumor is capable of propagating that tumor. Cancers that may follow this model include B-cell acute lymphoblastic leukemia[18] and malignant melanoma.[19] Most recently, advocates of both models concur in the literature that these cancer concepts are not mutually exclusive.[20,21]

TECHNIQUES USED TO STUDY CSCs

The ability to label cells according to specific cell surface markers using monoclonal antibodies combined with the capability to segregate specific populations based on their surface biomarker profile using fluorescence-activated cell sorting, significantly enhanced the study of purified CSC populations. Tumor-initiating cell assays performed on sorted cancer cell subpopulations do have their limitations; the act of segregating CSCs from the tumor bulk may have profound effects on cell-cell interactions and conversion of marker phenotype among CSC subpopulations (eg, CD133 has also been documented).[22]

Serial xenotransplantation in animal models is regarded as the gold standard to determine self-renewal capacity as well as tumor re-establishment for human tumor-initiating cells. Unfortunately, human-to-mouse xenotransplantation has its own limitations, including residual components of the murine immune system, lack of cross-species reactivity of cytokines, and variations in the murine versus human microenvironment. These variables can have very significant ramifications on experimental results with regard to estimations of CSC frequency.[23,24] For example, Quintana and colleagues[19] demonstrated that by using more immunodeficient mice, namely the NOD/SCID interleukin-2 receptor gamma chain null strain that lack natural killer cell activity, tumourigenic melanoma cells may comprise almost 25% of the bulk population instead of the 1 in 1 million, as previously shown.[25] This study in particular highlights limitations of xenotransplantation techniques with respect to estimating tumorigenic cell frequency and for extrapolating to the clinic for subsequent strategies for treatment.

HURDLES TOWARD A CURE FOR CML: THE CML STEM CELL

Successful cancer therapies must target the cancer cells that are responsible for disease maintenance and progression. According to traditional cancer therapies and the clonal evolution hypothesis, the entire tumor bulk is targeted. In CML in CP, the introduction of TKIs, such as IM and second-generation agents, DAS and NIL, which induce cytogenetic and molecular responses in most patients, has dramatically altered the natural history of the disease.[2,26,27] These agents are very effective in tumor debulking, and most patients with CML in CP achieve complete cytogenetic response (CCyR higher than 80% at 5 years), with progression-free survival and OS rates of more than 90%. Only 10% of CML CP cases achieve sustained complete molecular response (CMR) by 5 years. Therefore confirming that, although effective, IM fails to achieve full disease eradication.[2]

Following the original demonstration of the presence of a population of primitive, quiescent LSCs in all patients with CML in CP, which is thought to reside in the CD34+38-Lin- population, there is a solid foundation of evidence in support of CML following a CSC model.[28] We and others have demonstrated that CML stem and progenitor cells (eg, CD34+38-) are insensitive to induction of apoptosis by TKIs, although these agents exhibit potent antiproliferative effects.[29–33] This observation is paralleled by clinical observations that BCR-ABL–positive cells are still detectable by Q-RT-PCR within the primitive HSC compartment (CD34+38-) of patients with CML, despite continuous and successful IM treatment[34]; moreover, when TKIs are interrupted in patients in CMR, more than 50% of patients will show evidence of molecular relapse.[35] Mathematical models of the kinetics of the molecular response to IM also suggest that this drug inhibits production of differentiated leukemic cells, but does not deplete LSCs,[6] although this conclusion has been challenged in other models[7] and longer follow-up of patients on IM will be necessary to determine which model better fits the reality.

The CSC hypothesis proposes that targeting the elite subpopulation of CSCs responsible for recapitulating the tumor will yield successful therapy. Current evidence strongly suggests that the reason behind the inability of TKIs to cure CML in CP lies in the persistence of an LSC population whose survival is most likely dependent on unknown survival mechanisms inherent to the CML LSC. The real goal or absolute cure for CML should therefore involve drugs that will eliminate LSCs.

LSC RESISTANCE MECHANISMS

Oncogene addiction describes the dependency of tumor cells on a particular oncogene activity for growth and survival despite the presence of multiple genetic and epigenetic abnormalities.[36] This phenomenon provides the rationale to develop targeted therapies. In CML, BCR-ABL has been considered to play such a crucial role and this has led to development of TKI. Following the original observation of the persistence of LSC following TKI treatment, it was initially hypothesized that this could be explained by the persistence of BCR-ABL kinase activity in this subpopulation of cells; however, evidence is now growing to suggest that BCR-ABL kinase-dependent resistance mechanisms might not be sufficient to fully explain this phenomenon.

Mutations in the BCR-ABL kinase domain have been described in patients with CML in CP, but account for only 10% to 20% of cases that show suboptimal or failed response to IM[37] (fully reviewed in article 11). Furthermore, we have been unable to detect kinase domain mutations in CML LSCs that persist following prolonged TKI exposure in vitro (Hamilton and colleagues, unpublished data, 2011).

BCR-ABL transcripts are expressed at higher levels in LSCs as compared with more mature CML cells[30,38]; however, enhanced BCR-ABL inhibition with more potent TKIs is still unable to target quiescent LSCs, which remain viable and retain their clonogenic potential.[29,30,32] These observations are paralleled by clinical trial findings from front-line treatment of patients with CML in CP with more potent TKIs. Although DAS and NIL produce higher rates of CCyR and major molecular response at early time points, CMR rates are still low at about 10%, and extended follow-up is required to establish whether these agents eradicate CML stem cells. This is despite full inhibition of BCR-ABL kinase activity in most patients.[26,27]

Following reports that intracellular levels of IM in LSCs could be affected by either overexpression of the multidrug efflux transporter of the ATP-binding cassette (ABC) transporter family, MDR1, or reduced expression of the organic cation transporter hOCT-1,[38–40] the possibility that BCR-ABL kinase activity was not effectively inhibited in LSCs as the result of reduced intracellular drug accumulation has also been investigated.[41] For the efflux transporter ABCG2, a synthesis of experimental work suggests that although IM may be a substrate for ABCG2 at very low concentrations, at the concentrations that are relevant in the clinic, this drug acts as a potent ABCG2 inhibitor and would not therefore be effluxed from the cell.[41–43] Most recently, we have shown that CML CP CD34+ cells barely express MDR1 and inhibiting MDR1 does not result in increased efficacy of IM in vitro.[44] For hOCT-1, clinical observations suggest that high hOCT-1 activity is predictive of better response to IM.[45] Once again, at the stem cell level this transporter is barely expressed[46]; moreover, NIL concentration in CML cells, including LSCs, does not seem to be affected by drug transporters.[44,46] Therefore, the analysis of drug transporter expression and function on mature cells in patients with CML in CP before treatment might help in risk stratification and choice of TKI; however, it is unlikely to predict response at the stem cell level.

Although the presence of BCR-ABL kinase activity is necessary for leukemogenesis in vivo,[47] the activated ABL kinase is not sufficient on its own to reproduce the full disease spectrum in mice,[48] with multiple domains of BCR-ABL required to reproduce a CML-like disease.[49] In contrast to other oncogenes, BCR-ABL fails to confer self-renewal and stem cell potential to committed murine hematopoietic progenitor cells.[50] Recent collaborative research by several groups, including ours, has used a mouse model closely resembling human CML disease to show conclusively that leukemic long-term HSCs (LT-HSCs) are able to transplant disease, but that the BCR-ABL oncogene actually induces differentiation of the LT-HSCs and reduces their self-renewal potential. Leukemic LT-HSCs are preserved even when BCR-ABL expression is abrogated and can regenerate a CML-like disease on re-induction of BCR-ABL expression.[51] Finally, we have now shown that DAS, a multitargeted TKI that potently inhibits both BCR-ABL and SRC, rapidly (within 1–4 hours) initiates the process of irreversible apoptosis in 80% to 90% of bulk CD34+ CML CP cells; however, the remaining 10% to 20% of CML CP stem cells (CD34+38– and long-term culture-initiating cells) remain insensitive to extended drug exposure (to 12 days), to increased drug concentration (from 10–1000 nM), or to withdrawal of supplemental cytokines from the serum-free medium (Hamilton and colleagues, unpublished data, 2011). Taken together, these data argue strongly that inhibition of BCR-ABL kinase activity alone is insufficient to eradicate CML LSCs and suggest that BCR-ABL, or at least its kinase activity, might provide a proliferative advantage to CML LSCs, but does not represent the main molecular mechanism for their maintenance, which may instead be embedded within the key survival pathways that are inherent to normal stem cells.

As a consequence, one of the approaches currently being pursued to eradicate CML LSCs is to interfere with those pathways necessary for their maintenance (**Fig. 1**).

The concept of oncogene addiction as a passive dependence of tumor cells on particular oncogene activity has also been challenged by other investigators who have proposed an alternative model to explain cancer cell death on inactivation of a particular oncogene. This model, called 'oncogenic shock' states that, on inhibition of a particular oncogene, disruption of several signaling pathways happens, which preferentially leads to apoptosis as prosurvival signals are abrogated before proapoptotic signals.[52] The same investigators have shown that in a BCR-ABL–positive cell line, treatment with TKIs is associated with a transient imbalance between survival and apoptotic pathways, which results in tumor cell apoptosis.[53] It is obvious, therefore, that if survival or anti-apoptotic signaling is preserved or enhanced via alternative mechanisms at the time of BCR-ABL kinase inhibition, tumor cells will survive despite effective oncogene inhibition. This model emphasizes the role of those signaling pathways that remain active in LSCs at the time of TKI treatment. It has already been demonstrated that survival signals, such as those mediated by SRC kinases, can remain active following inhibition of BCR-ABL kinase activity by IM in CML cells.[54,55] A significant part of the current research in the CML community is exploring several signaling pathways for their role in CML LSC survival and is hoped to reveal alternative approaches to eradicate LSCs. Such approaches would likely consist of combining a TKI with a second inhibitor of survival signaling to more effectively shut down survival pathways active in LSCs (**Fig. 2**).

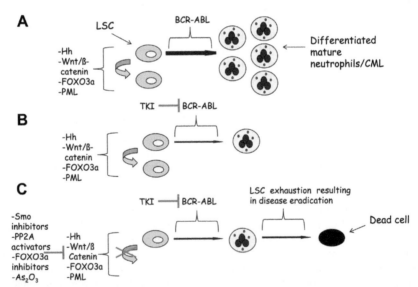

Fig. 1. Schematic diagram of the effects of tyrosine kinase inhibitors (TKIs) and potential agents targeting leukemic stem cell (LSC) self-maintenance in chronic myeloid leukemia (CML). (*A*) In untreated CML, LSCs are both preserved by self-maintenance pathways and prompted to proliferate/differentiate by the BCR-ABL oncogene giving rise to disease phenotype. (*B*) TKIs reduce the increased proliferation secondary to BCR-ABL and clear disease burden but fail to eradicate LSCs, with consequent risk of development of secondary resistance/relapse. (*C*) A strategy combining the debulking effects of TKI with agents targeting LSC maintenance could instead lead to LSC exhaustion and CML cure. As$_2$O$_3$, arsenic trioxide; FOXO3a, Forkhead O transcription factor 3; Hh, Hedgehog.

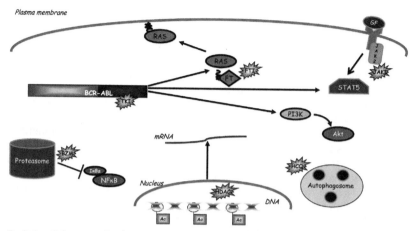

Fig. 2. Potential targets in chronic myeloid leukemia (CML), leukemic stem cells (LSC). BCR-ABL oncogene directly activates survival signaling pathways, such as Rat Sarcoma (RAS), PI3K/Akt, STAT5. Tyrosine kinase inhibitors (TKIs) act by directly inhibiting this mechanism; however, these and other survival/antiapoptotic pathways could still be kept active via alternative mechanisms, such as growth factors (GFs). Targeting these pathways together with TKIs could therefore provide a synergistic effect and eradicate LSCs. Farnesyltransferase (FT) inhibitors (FTI) specifically target RAS protein, inhibiting its prenylation and subsequent membrane anchoring necessary for its activation. JAK2 inhibitors (JAKI) block STAT5 activation via GF. Autophagy is a survival mechanism activated in CML LSCs following inhibition of BCR-ABL by TKI. Hydroxychloroquine (HCQ) specifically inhibits autophagy and is currently being investigated in patients with CML in chronic phase. Proteasome activity is increased in CML LSC. Bortezomib (BZM) is a proteasome inhibitor that has shown efficacy in CML LSCs and function via various mechanisms, such as reduced degradation of IκBα and subsequent cytoplasmic sequestration of transcription factor NFκB. Epigenetic modifiers, such as histone deacetylase inhibitors (HDACi), prevent removal of acetyl groups (Ac) from histones and keep chromatin in an active conformation, thus allowing ongoing transcription of tumor suppressor genes that would otherwise be silenced in CML cells. mRNA, messenger RNA.

TARGETING LSC MAINTENANCE TO INDUCE EXHAUSTION

The potential to target LSC self-renewal potential is an expanding area of research in CML. The embryonic morphogenic pathways Hedgehog (Hh) and Wnt/β-catenin have been shown to be active in CML and to play a significant role in CML LSC maintenance. In murine models, BCR-ABL–positive bone marrow progenitors lacking an active Hh pathway were reduced in number and showed reduced leukemogenic potential following transplantation into immunodeficient hosts.[56] This pathway seems to be active even in the presence of TKI and is specifically relevant to BCR-ABL–positive LSC maintenance and expansion, whereas normal LT-HSCs do not appear to be dependent on an active Hh pathway.[57] Smoothened (Smo) is a transmembrane receptor essential to transduce Hh signals and a potential target for therapy. Inhibition of Smo is able to specifically target the LSC pool, even in the presence of a mutated BCR-ABL kinase, in both mouse models and bone marrow from patients with CML.[56,57] LDE225 (Novartis) is a Smo antagonist that has already reached clinical development in solid tumors. It has been shown to target CML LSCs in combination with NIL.[58] Further in vivo studies in murine models are ongoing and it is hoped that this approach will be applied for improved treatment of CML in the near future.

The Wnt/β-catenin pathway is activated following binding of Wnt ligands to surface receptors, leading to nuclear localization of β-catenin and transcription of genes necessary for HSC self-renewal.[59] This pathway has been shown to be relevant for self-renewal of CML LSCs[60] and is now being investigated as a therapeutic target in CML.[61]

PP2A is a phosphatase with tumor suppressor activity present in normal stem and progenitor cells that appears to inhibit activation of β-catenin. Its activity is inhibited by SET, which is induced by BCR-ABL, leading to low or absent levels of PP2A in CML stem and progenitor cells. Restoration of PP2A activity in CML stem and progenitor cells leads to their apoptosis, and reduced clonogenic and in vivo leukemogenic potential.[62] The sphingosine analog, FTY720, is a powerful activator of PP2A and has been shown to induce apoptosis of CML progenitors, including the most quiescent population that is spared by TKI. These effects are thought to be secondary to suppression of signals regulated by PP2A via a BCR-ABL independent mechanism.[63]

More recently, the forkhead O transcription factor 3a (FOXO3a) has been identified to play a significant role in CML LSC maintenance/self-renewal. Naka and colleagues[64] have shown in a CML murine model that FOXO3a appears to be activated in LSCs by transforming growth factor beta (TGF-β) via inhibition of Akt. The TGF-β inhibitor, Ly364947, in combination with IM, led to improved survival of CML-bearing mice and reduced clonogenic potential of human CML LSCs. Our own data in primary human CML LSCs, with regard to FOXO activity and regulation, are highly complementary to the findings of Naka and colleagues.[65]

Another key feature of CML LSCs is their quiescence.[28] Inducing LSC proliferation would be anticipated to increase their sensitivity to many chemotherapeutic agents and in turn should lead to their exhaustion. This hypothesis resulted in studies of growth factors, such as granulocyte colony-stimulating factor (G-CSF), to stimulate quiescent CML LSCs into cell cycle. Despite promising in vitro results,[66,67] this approach failed to show any clinical benefit in a small pilot, phase II clinical study[68]; however, renewed interest in this concept has been raised by the recent understanding of a novel role for promyelocytic leukemia protein (PML) in CML. The PML gene, known to be involved in the development of acute promyelocytic leukemia, normally functions as a tumor suppressor and controls apoptosis and cell proliferation.[69] Although its loss of function has been described in several cancers, PML seems to be overexpressed in CML, particularly in CD34+ cells. In CML, PML seems to prevent quiescent LSCs from entering cell cycle. In murine LSCs, lack of PML then reversed their quiescence and enhanced their sensitivity to chemotherapy, leading to LSC exhaustion. Arsenic trioxide (As_2O_3) is known to target PML for degradation. In CML mouse models, the combination of As_2O_3 with standard cytotoxic chemotherapy achieved complete eradication of leukemia and induced higher levels of apoptosis in LSC from patients with CML.[70] Given that As_2O_3 is already in the clinic, it is hoped that a clinical trial of this drug in CML will happen in the near future.

TARGETING MULTIPLE SIGNALING PATHWAYS

Several molecular pathways commonly dysregulated in cancer have been shown to be relevant in CML and offer potential targets for therapies. As the number of putative pathways being investigated grows, evidence for their relevance is constantly changing. The focus here will be those pathways whose inhibition has been shown to be effective against LSCs from patients in CP.

The Rat Sarcoma (RAS) protein pathway has been shown to be activated in a variety of cancers, and is directly activated by BCR-ABL. Prenylation of RAS is necessary for its activation via anchoring of the protein to the plasma membrane. Prenylation is catalyzed by the enzyme farnesyltransferase (FT) and its inhibition can consequently lead to RAS inactivation. Several FT inhibitors (FTIs) have been tested in CML. Lonafarnib (Sarasar, Schering-Plough, Kenilworth, NJ, USA) as a single agent had minimal activity in patients with CML who have developed resistance to IM[71]; however, when used in combination with IM in vitro, it was shown to preferentially target primary quiescent CML LSCs.[72] More recently, an FTI developed by Bristol-Myers Squibb, BMS-214662, was demonstrated to have selective activity against quiescent LSC from patients with CML in CP in vitro, either as monotherapy or in combination with IM.[73] The mechanism of action against quiescent CML LSCs does not seem to be entirely mediated by FT inhibition, but by eliciting apoptosis via upregulation of PKCβ and Bax activation.[74] Currently, Bristol-Myers Squibb has no plans to further develop this molecule clinically; however, studies are under way to understand and enhance its proapoptotic activity in CML LSCs.

CML LSCs reside in a cytokine-rich environment; moreover, an autocrine loop has been demonstrated in CML primary cells for interleukin-3 (IL-3), G-CSF, and granulocyte-macrophage colony-stimulating factor.[75] Regardless of the mechanism of their production, it has been shown that growth factor (GF) signals can provide a resistance mechanism to CML LSCs, even in the presence of an inhibited BCR-ABL kinase.[76,77] As most of the hematopoietic GFs signal through the JAK/STAT pathway, JAK2 inhibitors (JAKI) are currently being investigated in CML experimental models with promising results.[78] As some of these JAKI are already in clinical development for myeloproliferative disorders, it is likely that if in vitro results are further validated, some of these compounds might reach clinical development in CML.

Abnormal epigenetic modifications have been found in a variety of hematological malignancies and are responsible for altered gene expression, leading to cancer cell survival and proliferation.[79] Histone deacetylase inhibitors (HDACi) are currently being developed in a variety of hematological malignancies and have also been tested in CML. In vitro data suggest that a combination of TKI and HDACi is able to target the LSC population selectively and effectively by inducing their apoptosis via a reduction of the MCL-1 antiapoptotic protein.[80] This has now been taken forward to a Phase I clinical trial of the HDACi LBH589 in combination with IM in patients with CML who have achieved at least a major cytogenetic response (MCyR), but still have detectable disease as measured by Q-RT-PCR.[81]

Proteasome inhibitors are known to induce apoptosis in a variety of hematological malignancies by several poorly understood mechanisms. BCR-ABL is associated with increased proteasome activity leading to the hypothesis that proteasome inhibition might be effective against CML LSCs that express high levels of the oncoprotein. Recent in vitro studies and mouse modeling have shown that bortezomib (Velcade, Millenium Pharmaceuticals, Cambridge, MA, USA), a proteasome inhibitor already in clinical use for myeloma and some subtypes of non-Hodgkin's lymphoma, targets primitive CML cells, but unfortunately at approximately the same 50% inhibition concentration as for normal CD34+ cells.[82] Given the toxicity of bortezomib to normal marrow CD34+ cells, it is likely that the initial clinical application of this drug to CML will be in patients with resistant and/or advanced disease.

Autophagy is a process activated in eukaryotic cells in response to homeostatic and stress conditions that allows cells to adapt to environmental/developmental signals by breaking down intracellular materials within lysosomes.[83] Depending on cellular context, autophagy can serve both as an alternative cell death mechanism or as a cell survival mechanism, whereby cells can adapt to starvation and evade cell death.[84] CML LSCs induce autophagy in response to TKIs, and suppression of autophagy, using either pharmacologic inhibitors (chloroquine or bafilomycin A1) or RNA interference of essential autophagy genes, enhances LSC death induced by TKIs.[85] These in vitro results have prompted the design of a Phase II trial of IM versus hydroxychloroquine with IM for patients with CML in MCyR with residual disease detectable by Q-RT-PCR, which has just started recruiting patients (www.mrc.ac.uk/Fundingopportunities/Grants/TSCRC/index.htm).

IMMUNOLOGIC APPROACHES

To date, the only curative treatment for CML is an alloSCT. In this clinical situation, cure is thought to be secondary to a graft-versus-leukemia effect (GVL).[86] The efficacy of donor lymphocyte infusion in inducing remission following relapse, or in the setting of minimal residual disease (MRD) post-alloSCT,[87] further validates this concept. The role of the immune response in CML eradication in the alloSCT setting has prompted further research into immunotherapeutic approaches for CML. Prompting an autologous immune response versus cells expressing specific tumor antigens is an approach currently being explored in a variety of malignancies, but is particularly attractive in CML, where it could be used to capitalize on the MRD status achieved following TKI treatment. The presence of a specific BCR-ABL fusion protein, which results in expression of novel unique epitopes, makes the development of immunologic therapies in CML technically possible. Several trials using vaccines against CML-specific peptides, either derived from the BCR-ABL protein or more generic to cancer, have been reported.[88–92] T-cell responses have been elicited in patients and a clinical effect with reduction of BCR-ABL Q-RT-PCR levels has been detected in most of these trials, predominantly in patients with less disease burden at the time of treatment. Larger, randomized trials are now needed to investigate this further.

Pharmacologic stimulation is another potential mechanism to harness the immune system in an attempt to eradicate CML. IFN-α has long been used in the treatment of CML and several other myeloproliferative disorders. Following the advent of TKI, its role in managing CML has been significantly reduced. Nonetheless, there is evidence that IFN-α may achieve long-term remission by targeting CML precursors immunologically, even permitting treatment discontinuation.[93] In particular, IFN-α has been shown to stimulate autologous T-cell responses versus specific tumor antigens and these immunologic responses correlated clinically with patients achieving long-lasting complete response.[94] In a recently published study, IFN-α was continued following IM discontinuation in 20 patients and resulted in durable molecular responses in 75% of patients, with some even achieving a deeper molecular response. These responses correlated with markers of immunologic activation and suggest that IFN-α has a significant single-agent activity in the context of prior IM/IFN-α combination therapy.[95]

SUMMARY

Treatment of CML in CP has changed significantly since the advent of TKIs, which are highly effective in reducing disease burden, but fail to achieve cure owing to LSC insensitivity to these agents. This could potentially lead to development of secondary resistance and has obvious implications in terms of compliance, adverse effects, and costs for patients who are required to commit to lifelong treatment. In the CML research community, a huge effort is currently being made to better understand the biology of LSCs in the hope that this will lead to the development of therapies targeted toward this highly resistant population. We believe that in the future, an approach combining a TKI to reduce disease burden and an agent to target the cancer stem cell population will be likely to achieve eradication of CML LSCs and hence CML cure.

ACKNOWLEDGMENTS

We would like to acknowledge our funding bodies Medical Research Council, UK (P.G.), Leukaemia&Lymphoma Research, UK (S.A.) and Cancer Research UK (T.L.H.).

REFERENCES

1. Sawyers CL. Chronic myeloid leukemia. N Engl J Med 1999;340(17):1330–40.
2. Druker BJ, Guilhot F, O'Brien SG, et al. Five-year follow-up of patients receiving imatinib for chronic myeloid leukemia. N Engl J Med 2006;355(23):2408–17.
3. Noens L, van Lierde MA, De Bock R, et al. Prevalence, determinants, and outcomes of nonadherence to imatinib therapy in patients with chronic myeloid leukemia: the ADAGIO study. Blood 2009;113(22):5401–11.
4. Marin D, Bazeos A, Mahon FX, et al. Adherence is the critical factor for achieving molecular responses in patients with chronic myeloid leukemia who achieve complete cytogenetic responses on imatinib. J Clin Oncol 2010;28(14):2381–8.
5. Ren R. Mechanisms of BCR-ABL in the pathogenesis of chronic myelogenous leukaemia. Nat Rev Cancer 2005;5(3):172–83.
6. Michor F, Hughes TP, Iwasa Y, et al. Dynamics of chronic myeloid leukaemia. Nature 2005;435(7046):1267–70.
7. Roeder I, Glauche I. Pathogenesis, treatment effects, and resistance dynamics in chronic myeloid leukemia—insights from mathematical model analyses. J Mol Med 2008;86(1):17–27.
8. Dick JE. Stem cell concepts renew cancer research. Blood 2008;112(13): 4793–807.
9. Becker AJ, McCulloch EA, Till JE. Cytological demonstration of the clonal nature of spleen colonies derived from transplanted mouse marrow cells. Nature 1963; 197:452–4.
10. Nowell PC. The clonal evolution of tumor cell populations. Science 1976; 194(4260):23–8.
11. Lapidot T, Sirard C, Vormoor J, et al. A cell initiating human acute myeloid leukaemia after transplantation into SCID mice. Nature 1994;367(6464):645–8.
12. Bonnet D, Dick JE. Human acute myeloid leukemia is organized as a hierarchy that originates from a primitive hematopoietic cell. Nat Med 1997;3(7):730–7.
13. Clarke MF, Dick JE, Dirks PB, et al. Cancer stem cells—perspectives on current status and future directions: AACR Workshop on cancer stem cells. Cancer Res 2006;66(19):9339–44.
14. Misaghian N, Ligresti G, Steelman LS, et al. Targeting the leukemic stem cell: the Holy Grail of leukemia therapy. Leukemia 2009;23(1):25–42.
15. Lane SW, Scadden DT, Gilliland DG. The leukemic stem cell niche: current concepts and therapeutic opportunities. Blood 2009;114(6):1150–7.
16. Schatton T, Frank NY, Frank MH. Identification and targeting of cancer stem cells. Bioessays 2009;31(10):1038–49.
17. Frank NY, Schatton T, Frank MH. The therapeutic promise of the cancer stem cell concept. J Clin Invest 2010;120(1):41–50.
18. Hong D, Gupta R, Ancliff P, et al. Initiating and cancer-propagating cells in TEL-AML1-associated childhood leukemia. Science 2008;319(5861):336–9.
19. Quintana E, Shackleton M, Sabel MS, et al. Efficient tumour formation by single human melanoma cells. Nature 2008;456(7222):593–8.
20. Shackleton M, Quintana E, Fearon ER, et al. Heterogeneity in cancer: cancer stem cells versus clonal evolution. Cell 2009;138(5):822–9.

21. Dick JE. Looking ahead in cancer stem cell research. Nat Biotechnol 2009;27(1): 44–6.
22. Jaksch M, Munera J, Bajpai R, et al. Cell cycle-dependent variation of a CD133 epitope in human embryonic stem cell, colon cancer, and melanoma cell lines. Cancer Res 2008;68(19):7882–6.
23. Kelly PN, Dakic A, Adams JM, et al. Tumor growth need not be driven by rare cancer stem cells. Science 2007;317(5836):337.
24. Kennedy JA, Barabe F, Poeppl AG, et al. Comment on "Tumor growth need not be driven by rare cancer stem cells". Science 2007;318(5857):1722 [author reply: 1722].
25. Schatton T, Murphy GF, Frank NY, et al. Identification of cells initiating human melanomas. Nature 2008;451(7176):345–9.
26. Cortes JE, Jones D, O'Brien S, et al. Nilotinib as front-line treatment for patients with chronic myeloid leukemia in early chronic phase. J Clin Oncol 2010;28(3): 392–7.
27. Cortes JE, Jones D, O'Brien S, et al. Results of dasatinib therapy in patients with early chronic-phase chronic myeloid leukemia. J Clin Oncol 2010;28(3): 398–404.
28. Holyoake T, Jiang X, Eaves C, et al. Isolation of a highly quiescent subpopulation of primitive leukemic cells in chronic myeloid leukemia. Blood 1999;94(6): 2056–64.
29. Jorgensen HG, Allan EK, Jordanides NE, et al. Nilotinib exerts equipotent antiproliferative effects to imatinib and does not induce apoptosis in CD34+ CML cells. Blood 2007;109(9):4016–9.
30. Copland M, Hamilton A, Elrick LJ, et al. Dasatinib (BMS-354825) targets an earlier progenitor population than imatinib in primary CML but does not eliminate the quiescent fraction. Blood 2006;107(11):4532–9.
31. Graham SM, Jorgensen HG, Allan E, et al. Primitive, quiescent, Philadelphia-positive stem cells from patients with chronic myeloid leukemia are insensitive to STI571 in vitro. Blood 2002;99(1):319–25.
32. Konig H, Holtz M, Modi H, et al. Enhanced BCR-ABL kinase inhibition does not result in increased inhibition of downstream signaling pathways or increased growth suppression in CML progenitors. Leukemia 2008;22(4):748–55.
33. Konig H, Holyoake TL, Bhatia R. Effective and selective inhibition of chronic myeloid leukemia primitive hematopoietic progenitors by the dual Src/Abl kinase inhibitor SKI-606. Blood 2008;111(4):2329–38.
34. Chu S, Lin A, McDonald T, et al. Persistence of leukemia stem cells in chronic myelogenous leukemia patients in complete cytogenetic remission on imatinib treatment for 5 years. Blood 2008;112(11):79.
35. Mahon F, Rea F, Guilhot F, et al. Discontinuation of imatinib therapy after achieving a molecular response in chronic myeloid leukemia patients. Blood 2009;114(22): [abstract: 859].
36. Weinstein IB, Joe A. Oncogene addiction. Cancer Res 2008;68(9):3077–80 [discussion: 3080].
37. Hughes T, Saglio G, Martinelli G, et al. Responses and disease progression in CML-CP patients treated with nilotinib after imatinib failure appear to be affected by the BCR-ABL mutation status and types. Blood 2007;110(11): 101a.
38. Jiang X, Zhao Y, Smith C, et al. Chronic myeloid leukemia stem cells possess multiple unique features of resistance to BCR-ABL targeted therapies. Leukemia 2007;21(5):926–35.

39. Mahon FX, Belloc F, Lagarde V, et al. MDR1 gene overexpression confers resistance to imatinib mesylate in leukemia cell line models. Blood 2003;101(6):2368–73.

40. Engler JR, Frede A, Saunders VA, et al. Chronic myeloid leukemia CD34+ cells have reduced uptake of imatinib due to low OCT-1 activity. Leukemia 2010;24(4):765–70.

41. Jordanides NE, Jorgensen HG, Holyoake TL, et al. Functional ABCG2 is overexpressed on primary CML CD34+ cells and is inhibited by imatinib mesylate. Blood 2006;108(4):1370–3.

42. Houghton PJ, Germain GS, Harwood FC, et al. Imatinib mesylate is a potent inhibitor of the ABCG2 (BCRP) transporter and reverses resistance to topotecan and SN-38 in vitro. Cancer Res 2004;64(7):2333–7.

43. Burger H, van Tol H, Boersma AW, et al. Imatinib mesylate (STI571) is a substrate for the breast cancer resistance protein (BCRP)/ABCG2 drug pump. Blood 2004;104(9):2940–2.

44. Hatziieremia S, Jordanides NE, Holyoake TL, et al. Inhibition of MDR1 does not sensitize primitive chronic myeloid leukemia CD34+ cells to imatinib. Exp Hematol 2009;37(6):692–700.

45. White DL, Saunders VA, Dang P, et al. Most CML patients who have a suboptimal response to imatinib have low OCT-1 activity: higher doses of imatinib may overcome the negative impact of low OCT-1 activity. Blood 2007;110(12):4064–72.

46. Davies A, Jordanides NE, Giannoudis A, et al. Nilotinib concentration in cell lines and primary CD34(+) chronic myeloid leukemia cells is not mediated by active uptake or efflux by major drug transporters. Leukemia 2009;23(11):1999–2006.

47. Zhang X, Ren R. Bcr-Abl efficiently induces a myeloproliferative disease and production of excess interleukin-3 and granulocyte-macrophage colony-stimulating factor in mice: a novel model for chronic myelogenous leukemia. Blood 1998;92(10):3829–40.

48. Gross AW, Zhang X, Ren R. Bcr-Abl with an SH3 deletion retains the ability To induce a myeloproliferative disease in mice, yet c-Abl activated by an SH3 deletion induces only lymphoid malignancy. Mol Cell Biol 1999;19(10):6918–28.

49. Johnson KJ, Griswold IJ, O'Hare T, et al. A BCR-ABL mutant lacking direct binding sites for the GRB2, CBL and CRKL adapter proteins fails to induce leukemia in mice. PLoS One 2009;4(10):e7439.

50. Huntly BJ, Shigematsu H, Deguchi K, et al. MOZ-TIF2, but not BCR-ABL, confers properties of leukemic stem cells to committed murine hematopoietic progenitors. Cancer Cell 2004;6(6):587–96.

51. Schemionek M, Elling C, Steidl U, et al. BCR-ABL enhances differentiation of long-term repopulating hematopoietic stem cells. Blood 2010;115(16):3185–95.

52. Sharma SV, Fischbach MA, Haber DA, et al. "Oncogenic shock": explaining oncogene addiction through differential signal attenuation. Clin Cancer Res 2006;12(14 Pt 2):4392s–5s.

53. Sharma SV, Gajowniczek P, Way IP, et al. A common signaling cascade may underlie "addiction" to the Src, BCR-ABL, and EGF receptor oncogenes. Cancer Cell 2006;10(5):425–35.

54. Hu Y, Swerdlow S, Duffy TM, et al. Targeting multiple kinase pathways in leukemic progenitors and stem cells is essential for improved treatment of Ph+ leukemia in mice. Proc Natl Acad Sci U S A 2006;103(45):16870–5.

55. Donato NJ, Wu JY, Stapley J, et al. Imatinib mesylate resistance through BCR-ABL independence in chronic myelogenous leukemia. Cancer Res 2004;64(2):672–7.

56. Zhao C, Chen A, Jamieson CH, et al. Hedgehog signalling is essential for maintenance of cancer stem cells in myeloid leukaemia. Nature 2009;458(7239): 776–9.

57. Dierks C, Beigi R, Guo GR, et al. Expansion of Bcr-Abl-positive leukemic stem cells is dependent on Hedgehog pathway activation. Cancer Cell 2008;14(3): 238–49.

58. Irvine D, Zhang B, Allan E, et al. Combination of the hedgehog pathway inhibitor LDE225 and nilotinib eliminates chronic myeloid leukemia stem and progenitor cells. Blood 2009;114(22): [abstract: 1428].

59. Nusse R. Wnt signaling and stem cell control. Cell Res 2008;18(5):523–7.

60. Hu Y, Chen Y, Douglas L, et al. beta-Catenin is essential for survival of leukemic stem cells insensitive to kinase inhibition in mice with BCR-ABL-induced chronic myeloid leukemia. Leukemia 2009;23(1):109–16.

61. Peterson L, Turbiak A, Giannola D, et al. Wnt-pathway directed compound targets blast crisis and chronic phase CML leukemia stem progenitors. Blood 2009; 114(22): [abstract: 2168].

62. Neviani P, Santhanam R, Trotta R, et al. The tumor suppressor PP2A is functionally inactivated in blast crisis CML through the inhibitory activity of the BCR/ABL-regulated SET protein. Cancer Cell 2005;8(5):355–68.

63. Neviani P, Santhanam R, Ma Y, et al. Activation of PP2A by FTY720 inhibits survival and self-renewal of the Ph(+) chronic myelogenous leukemia (CML) CD34+/CD38– stem cell through the simultaneous suppression of BCR/ABL and BCR/ABL– independent signals. Blood 2008;112(11): [abstract: 189].

64. Naka K, Hoshii T, Muraguchi T, et al. TGF-beta-FOXO signalling maintains leukaemia-initiating cells in chronic myeloid leukaemia. Nature 2010;463(7281): 676–80.

65. Pellicano F, Huntly BJ, Holyoake TL. Investigation of the role of FOXO in TKI-induced G1 arrest as potential targets in CML stem/progenitor cell eradication. Abstract presented at ESH-EHA Scientific Workshop Leukemic and Cancer Stem Cells. Mandelieu (France), April 3–5, 2009.

66. Jorgensen HG, Copland M, Allan EK, et al. Intermittent exposure of primitive quiescent chronic myeloid leukemia cells to granulocyte-colony stimulating factor in vitro promotes their elimination by imatinib mesylate. Clin Cancer Res 2006; 12(2):626–33.

67. Holtz M, Forman SJ, Bhatia R. Growth factor stimulation reduces residual quiescent chronic myelogenous leukemia progenitors remaining after imatinib treatment. Cancer Res 2007;67(3):1113–20.

68. Drummond MW, Heaney N, Kaeda J, et al. A pilot study of continuous imatinib vs pulsed imatinib with or without G-CSF in CML patients who have achieved a complete cytogenetic response. Leukemia 2009;23(6):1199–201.

69. Salomoni P, Pandolfi PP. The role of PML in tumor suppression. Cell 2002;108(2): 165–70.

70. Ito K, Bernardi R, Morotti A, et al. PML targeting eradicates quiescent leukaemia-initiating cells. Nature 2008;453(7198):1072–8.

71. Borthakur G, Kantarjian H, Daley G, et al. Pilot study of lonafarnib, a farnesyl transferase inhibitor, in patients with chronic myeloid leukemia in the chronic or accelerated phase that is resistant or refractory to imatinib therapy. Cancer 2006;106(2):346–52.

72. Jorgensen HG, Allan EK, Graham SM, et al. Lonafarnib reduces the resistance of primitive quiescent CML cells to imatinib mesylate in vitro. Leukemia 2005;19(7): 1184–91.

73. Copland DA, Wertheim MS, Armitage WJ, et al. The clinical time-course of experimental autoimmune uveoretinitis using topical endoscopic fundal imaging with histologic and cellular infiltrate correlation. Invest Ophthalmol Vis Sci 2008; 49(12):5458–65.

74. Pellicano F, Copland M, Jorgensen HG, et al. BMS-214662 induces mitochondrial apoptosis in chronic myeloid leukemia (CML) stem/progenitor cells, including CD34+38– cells, through activation of protein kinase Cbeta. Blood 2009; 114(19):4186–96.

75. Jiang X, Lopez A, Holyoake T, et al. Autocrine production and action of IL-3 and granulocyte colony-stimulating factor in chronic myeloid leukemia. Proc Natl Acad Sci U S A 1999;96(22):12804–9.

76. Hiwase DK, White DL, Powell JA, et al. Blocking cytokine signaling along with intense Bcr-Abl kinase inhibition induces apoptosis in primary CML progenitors. Leukemia 2010;24(4):771–8.

77. Wang Y, Cai D, Brendel C, et al. Adaptive secretion of granulocyte-macrophage colony-stimulating factor (GM-CSF) mediates imatinib and nilotinib resistance in BCR/ABL+ progenitors via JAK-2/STAT-5 pathway activation. Blood 2007; 109(5):2147–55.

78. Samanta A, Chakraborty S, Sun X, et al. Jak2 phosphorylates Tyr 177 of Bcr-Abl activating the Ras and PI-3 kinase pathways and maintains functional levels of Bcr-Abl in chronic myelogenous leukemia. Blood 2009;114(22): [abstract: 39].

79. Mercurio C, Minucci S, Pelicci PG. Histone deacetylases and epigenetic therapies of hematological malignancies. Pharm Res 2010;62(1):18–34.

80. Zhang B, Campbell Strauss A, Chu S, et al. Effective targeting of quiescent CML stem cells by histone deacetylase inhibitors in combination with imatinib mesylate. Blood 2009;114(22): [abstract: 190].

81. Bhatia R, Snyder D, Lin A, et al. A phase I study of the HDAC inhibitor LBH589 in combination with imatinib for patients with CML in cytogenetic remission with residual disease detectable by Q-PCR [abstract: 2194]. Blood 2009;114(22).

82. Heaney NB, Pellicano F, Zhang B, et al. Bortezomib induces apoptosis in primitive chronic myeloid leukemia cells including LTC-IC and NOD/SCID repopulating cells. Blood 2010;115(11):2241–50.

83. Klionsky DJ. Autophagy: from phenomenology to molecular understanding in less than a decade. Nat Rev Mol Cell Biol 2007;8(11):931–7.

84. Lum JJ, Bauer DE, Kong M, et al. Growth factor regulation of autophagy and cell survival in the absence of apoptosis. Cell 2005;120(2):237–48.

85. Bellodi C, Lidonnici MR, Hamilton A, et al. Targeting autophagy potentiates tyrosine kinase inhibitor-induced cell death in Philadelphia chromosome-positive cells, including primary CML stem cells. J Clin Invest 2009;119(5):1109–23.

86. Kolb HJ, Schattenberg A, Goldman JM, et al. Graft-versus-leukemia effect of donor lymphocyte transfusions in marrow grafted patients. Blood 1995;86(5): 2041–50.

87. Kolb HJ, Mittermuller J, Clemm C, et al. Donor leukocyte transfusions for treatment of recurrent chronic myelogenous leukemia in marrow transplant patients. Blood 1990;76(12):2462–5.

88. Rojas JM, Knight K, Wang L, et al. Clinical evaluation of BCR-ABL peptide immunisation in chronic myeloid leukaemia: results of the EPIC study. Leukemia 2007; 21(11):2287–95.

89. Jain N, Reuben JM, Kantarjian H, et al. Synthetic tumor-specific breakpoint peptide vaccine in patients with chronic myeloid leukemia and minimal residual disease: a phase 2 trial. Cancer 2009;115(17):3924–34.

90. Smith BD, Kasamon YL, Kowalski J, et al. K562/GM-CSF immunotherapy reduces tumor burden in chronic myeloid leukemia patients with residual disease on imatinib mesylate. Clin Cancer Res 2010;16(1):338–47.
91. Maslak PG, Dao T, Gomez M, et al. A pilot vaccination trial of synthetic analog peptides derived from the BCR-ABL breakpoints in CML patients with minimal disease. Leukemia 2008;22(8):1613–6.
92. Li Z, Qiao Y, Liu B, et al. Combination of imatinib mesylate with autologous leukocyte-derived heat shock protein and chronic myelogenous leukemia. Clin Cancer Res 2005;11(12):4460–8.
93. Kantarjian HM, O'Brien S, Cortes JE, et al. Complete cytogenetic and molecular responses to interferon-alpha-based therapy for chronic myelogenous leukemia are associated with excellent long-term prognosis. Cancer 2003; 97(4):1033–41.
94. Molldrem JJ, Lee PP, Wang C, et al. Evidence that specific T lymphocytes may participate in the elimination of chronic myelogenous leukemia. Nat Med 2000; 6(9):1018–23.
95. Burchert A, Muller MC, Kostrewa P, et al. Sustained molecular response with interferon alfa maintenance after induction therapy with imatinib plus interferon alfa in patients with chronic myeloid leukemia. J Clin Oncol 2010;28(8):1429–35.

The Biology of Chronic Myelogenous Leukemia Progression: Who, What, Where, and Why?

Jerald P. Radich, MD

KEYWORDS

- Chronic myeloid leukemia • Blast crisis • Progression
- Genetic instability

Tyrosine kinase inhibitors (TKIs) have vastly and irreversibly changed the course of chronic myelogenous leukemia (CML) treatment. The vast majority of these CML cases present in chronic phase, and the use of TKI can yield complete cytogenetic remissions, and long-term progression-free survival, in approximately 80% of cases. Unfortunately, patients sometimes present in advanced-phase CML (accelerated or blast phase), and for these cases treatments with TKI alone are ineffective. Moreover, the approximately 10% of chronic-phase cases that have initial resistance to TKI therapy, as well as about another 10% who become resistant to primary and secondary TKI therapy, are likely to progress to advanced-phase disease.[1,2] Thus, an understanding of the process of CML progression may (1) offer new targets for therapy; (2) allow us to develop prognostic markers to predict patients at high risk of progression; and (3) tell us something about the "biological clock" that drives progression in CML and (hopefully) other malignancies.

Recently several outstanding reviews of CML progression have been published, and it is not the author's intention to simply recapitulate them here.[3,4] Rather, this article takes a different approach to looking at CML, in the spirit of solving a crime or a mystery: the author asks who, what, where, and why? With enough evidence, one can then try to infer *how* progression might be treated.

WHO PROGRESSES?

There are several classification models of CML (**Table 1**) that rely on clinical and pathologic features (blast counts, cytogenetics, splenomegaly, and so forth).[5] The most recent change in classification was introduced by the World Health Organization,

Clinical Research Division, Fred Hutchinson Cancer Research Center, Seattle, WA, USA
E-mail address: jradich@fhcrc.org

Hematol Oncol Clin N Am 25 (2011) 967–980
doi:10.1016/j.hoc.2011.09.002

Table 1
Classification schemes in CML, accelerated and blast phases

Features	Sokol	IBMT	MDA	WHO
Blast %	≥5%	≥10%	≥15%	10%–19%
Clonal evolution?	Yes	Yes	Yes	Yes
Platelet count	Increased	Decreased	Decreased	Increased/decreased
Blast count (BC)	≥30%	≥30%	≥30%	≥20%

An abbreviated summary of classification schemes for CML. The greatest variation is defining the transition from chronic to accelerated phase (top 3 rows). The differences in the definition of blast crisis focus on the percentage of blast counts in the bone marrow or peripheral blood. Definitions: "Blast %" refers to peripheral blood or bone marrow; "clonal evolution" are secondary chromosomal changes in addition to the Ph; "Platelet count" refers to significant changes (eg, >1 × 10^{12}/L) while on therapy.

Abbreviations: IBMT, International Bone Marrow Transplantation; MDA, MD Anderson; WHO, World Health Organization.

which decreased the percentage of blast counts needed to qualify for acute leukemia from 30% to 20%. That being said, it is unlikely that there is any biological difference in an "accelerated-phase" case with 17% blasts and a "blast-crisis" case with 20% blasts. Indeed, gene expression studies have shown that there is little difference between accelerated and blast crisis; rather, the biology of progression appears at the critical transition from chronic phase to accelerated phase.[6] At that point, the proverbial horse is out of the barn.

In the days before "curative" therapy for CML (transplantation and now, potentially, TKI), all cases of chronic phase eventually progressed, with the median time from diagnosis to accelerated phase of around 4 years. From this point, further progression to blast crisis took on the order of months. In the Western world, CML is generally diagnosed in chronic phase, and progression is limited to those cases resistant to TKI therapy. However, in Asia the disease appears to occur less frequently but in a younger population, and some surveys suggest that response to therapy is worse compared with Western countries, though it is unclear as to what contribution access and patterns of care, and biology, play in this pattern.[7]

There appears to be a relationship of progression and resistance to TKI therapy. The most obvious link is the association of response with phase of disease. Complete cytogenetic response (CCyR) to imatinib is the rule in chronic-phase CML; in blast crisis there is an initial response in most patients, but a CCyR is relatively unusual, and if it occurs is generally short-lived. TKI resistance is often mediated by point mutations in the Abl tyrosine kinase domain, which may be associated with a relief of kinase inhibition, or may alter the signaling pathways of BCR-ABL.[8–10] Resistance associated with Abl mutations is uncommon in newly diagnosed chronic-phase CML, and increases in frequency as time from diagnosis, or phase, progresses.[2,9] Indeed, point mutations can be found in blast-crisis samples never exposed to TKIs.[10]

The acquisition of point mutations may result from the genetic instability associated with BCR-ABL[11] (see later discussion). Point mutations have been found in the CD34+ cells derived from CCyR patients.[12,13] Thus, even in the context of an excellent response, residual CML stem cells remain, and while on therapy there is either an expansion of a resistant clone or the development of a clone. Lastly, gene expression arrays were performed on CML patients, who achieved a CCyR but then had a relapse into clinical chronic phase, most with point mutations. Many of these cases had gene expression profiles more similar to advanced-phase disease.[6]

WHAT IS PROGRESSION?

Blast crisis is fundamentally different to chronic phase in many aspects. By definition, accelerated phase and blast crisis are associated with other chromosomal structural changes (**Table 2**). Often, progression is associated with additional chromosomal abnormalities that involve the Ph. "Double" Ph are seen in more than 30% of blast-crisis patients.[14] Additional loss of chromosome 9 (der 9) occurs in 5% to 10% of chronic-phase patients; there are some data that these cases respond poorly to interferon, likely because this deletion eliminates critical interferon receptor genes. It is not clear whether the der 9 abnormality affects prognosis for patients treated with imatinib or transplantation.[15,16]

Progression appears to be associated with an increase in BCR-ABL activity. The aberrant cellular activities of BCR-ABL have been well chronicled (reviewed nicely in Ref.[3]), including increased proliferation through the activation of RAS[17]; increased transcriptional activity via STAT recruitment[18,19]; decreases in apoptosis through activation of PI(3)K/AKT[20]; and changes in adhesion binding to actin with phosphorylation to cytoskeletal proteins.[21] Blast phase is accompanied by an increase in both BCR-ABL mRNA and protein level. Although the levels are modestly increased (~ 3 fold for both message and protein), they are associated with an increase in activation of signaling (as evidenced by increased Crkl phosphorylation) and in vitro changes of clonality, growth factor independence, proliferation, and block in apoptosis.[22–24] In mouse models, cells constructed to produce more BCR-ABL have a more rapid tumor development.[23] Because BCR-ABL level is associated with progression, a logical question is whether this phenomenon also plays a role in imatinib resistance. A model using cell lines cultured in imatinib to develop resistance suggested high BCR-ABL was associated with a shorter time to the development of Abl point mutations.

Table 2
Genetic lesions found in advanced-phase CML

Genetic Lesion	Mechanism	Functional Effects
Chromosomal		
BCR-ABL	Amplification	Myriad
NUP98-HOXA9, AML1-EVI1	Translocation	Differentiation
TP53	Deletion	Tumor suppressor
P16/ARF	Deletion	Proliferation
Point mutations		
TP53	Point mutation	Tumor suppressor
Expression/translation		
CEBPA	Translational block	Differentiation
hnENPE2	Increased expression	Differentiation
PP2A	Inhibition by SET	Tumor suppressor
Bcl2	Increased expression	Apoptosis
FOXO3A	Decreased expression	Apoptosis
JunB	Decreased expression	Transcriptional regulation
WT1	Increased expression	Proliferation
BMI1	Expression	Proliferation

This table represents a sampling of the genes implicated in progression, and the best approximation of the pathways involved.

Conversely, a model of human CD34$^+$ cells transduced with BCR-ABL found that high BCR-ABL expression was associated with increased sensitivity to imatinib, suggesting that such cells were "addicted" to high levels of BCR-ABL.[23,24] Of note is that the mechanism of increased BCR-ABL mRNA and protein levels in progressive disease is unclear, while because some cases of blast crisis have multiple copies of the Ph chromosome, such abnormalities are not the rule.

Increased BCR-ABL activity is also associated with a change in mRNA processing.[25] The most notable changes associated with progression involve alternative splicing glycogen synthase kinase 3B (GSK3B).[26] GSK3B is involved in the inactivation of β-catenin, and the aberrant splicing is thought to inhibit proper functioning, allowing β-catenin to activate transcription and thus increase self-renewal pathways. In addition, aberrant splicing of Ikaros (IKZF1) has been described in cases of lymphoid blast crisis, thus making the functional depletion of IKZF1 through deletion or missplicing quite common in that disease.[27] In addition, studies of the RNA-binding proteins Lin28 and Lin28B have been shown to be elevated in CML progression. LIN28B is 1 of the 4 genes (with OCT4, NONOG, and SOX2) that can "reprogram" human fibroblast to a pluripotent state.[28] Lin28/28B block let-7 miRNA processing into mature miRNAs; given that the let-7 family is repressed in human malignancies, the elevation of Lin28B in blast crisis is likely functionally significant.[29]

Is Genetic Instability the Key Driver or Progression?

The main functional changes that occur with progression of CML are marked changes in proliferation, differentiation, apoptosis, and adhesion.[30,31] These functional changes accompanying progression are accompanied by profound changes in treatment response. But what drives progression?

There is growing evidence that BCR-ABL itself is a direct cause of the genetic instability seen in progression. While the contributions of these pathways in the initiation CML are logical, it is not clear that these pathways alone drive progression from chronic phase to advanced phase. However, insights that BCR-ABL causes genetic instability[32] may prove to be a unifying theme in starting the basis for progression at the very beginning of CML. When considering the effect of BCR-ABL on genetic instability, one must confront a seeming paradox: cell lines with activated tyrosine kinases, such as BCR-ABL, accumulate more DNA damage than those cell lines without activated kinases, yet these cell lines also repair the DNA damage faster.[33,34] The combination of more DNA damage and repair activity may lead to less accurate repair. As BCR-ABL upregulates antiapoptosis genes BCL2 and BCL-XI, thus causing G2/M delay, cells accumulate DNA damage but are not targeted for cell death.[34] It also appears that BCR-ABL directly causes DNA damage by increasing reactive oxygen species (ROS)[35]; ROS leads to DNA base-pair transversions (GC→TA) and transitions (GC→AT). Thus, unbridled BCR-ABL activity may contribute to the genetic instability leading to chromosomal aberrations, mutations, and changes in gene expression that cause progression.

Genetic Structural Changes

Chromosomal changes in addition to the Ph are the norm in blast crisis. Isochromosome i(17q) is a relatively common occurrence (~20% of cases of blast-crisis cases), and this is likely associated with progression, as it means the loss of a copy of the p53 tumor suppressor gene. However, the remaining p53 allele does not seem to be mutated in these cases, so a direct link of p53 inactivation and progress to blast crisis is not so clear,[36] though the reduction of the total cellular p53 level may upset the integration of genetic repair and apoptosis and thus contribute to progression.[37]

Alternatively, there may be critical but yet unknown genes on 17q contributing to progression. Trisomy 8 is also common in blast crisis (~40%), which is interesting because Myc is located at 8q24. There are several lines of evidence linking MYC to progression. In vitro inhibition of c-Myc with antisense oligonucleotides, or dominant-negative constructs, can inhibit BCR-ABL transformation or leukemogenesis.[38] Myc is often overexpressed in blast crisis compared with chronic phase[6,39]; whereas in acute myelogenous leukemia (AML) cases with trisomy 8, c-Myc is downregulated, but other genes on chromosome 8 are upregulated.[40] However, trisomy 8 is a common feature of cases of CML that exhibit clonal evolution Ph-negative cells while in a CCyR (see later discussion). These cases of Ph-negative, trisomy 8 appear to have a benign course, suggesting that trisomy 8 may not be leukemogenic.[41]

Translocations of known oncogenes in blast crisis occur relatively rarely (<5%). The most notable of these recurrent translocations are t(3;21) and t(7;11), involving the AML-1/EVI-1 and NUP98/HOXA9 genes, respectively.[42,43] Evi-1 and HOXA9 are both transcription factors, and their aberrant expression in the context of these fusion proteins causes differentiation arrest in the case of AML-1/EVI-1, and increased proliferation in the case of NUP98/HOXAP. In mouse models, BCR-ABL and AML-1/EVI-1 coexpression creates a disease produces a picture of myeloid leukemia, whereas mice transplanted with cells transfected with NUP98/HOXAP develop a myeloproliferative disease that evolves into an acute leukemia.[44,45] Recently it was shown that NUP98-HOXA9 increased the expression of the RNA binding protein Musashi 2 (Msi2), which in turn repressed the Numb expression, involved in the control of Notch signaling. Msi2 was found to be overexpressed in blast-crisis cases compared with chronic phase; moreover, increased Msi2 expression was found to be associated with poorer survival in all phases of CML following allogeneic transplantation.[46]

Disruption of Critical Pathways in Progression

Activation of the MAPK proliferation pathway is central in myeloid leukemia (BCR-ABL in CML, RAS, FLT3, kit mutations in AML). Thus, it is not surprising that RAS and FLT3 mutations are rare in CML progression, because their activation would not add to the selective advantage already conferred by BCR-ABL.[47] The tumor suppressor p53, inactivated in many solid tumors, is occasionally involved in blast crisis (~20%–30%); it is not known if there are aberrations in genes involved in p53-mediated function.[48] In lymphoid blast crisis (but not myeloid), a homozygous deletion of exon 2 of INK4A/ARF occurs commonly (~50%).[49] This deletion eliminates both p16 and p19, two proteins that normally check G1/S cell cycle progression and upregulate p53.

The activity of the tumor suppressor PP2A may be involved in the pathogenesis of CML progression and may provide a new drug target. PP2A activity is involved in regulating proliferation, survival, and differentiation, and is involved in the proteosomal degradation of BCR-ABL. Increasing BCR-ABL levels (induced in vitro or in human leukemia) increases the expression of the phosphoprotein SET, a negative regulator of PP2A.[6,50] Thus, progression may set up a feedback loop whereby increasing BCR-ABL increases SET, decreasing PP2A, which further ensures the persistence of BCR-ABL. In in vitro and mouse models, restoration of PP2A activity by the activator forskolin appeared to decrease BCR-ABL leukemic potential, thus suggesting a potential therapeutic target to arrest or regress CML progression.[50]

A block in myeloid differentiation occurs in progression, contributing to the accumulation of immature blasts. A search for mutations differentiation genes has been relatively unrewarding. For example, the CCAAT/enhancer binding protein α (CEBPA) is a member of the basic leucine zipper family of transcription factors essential to the control of granulocytic differentiation, regulating several genes necessary for orderly differentiation, including CSFR3. Inhibition of CEBPA in t(8;21) AML occurs through repression on CEBPA by the fusion AML1-ETO protein. In blast-crisis CML, high levels of BCR-ABL induce the MAPK phosphorylation of the poly(rC) binding protein hnENPE2, which then causes the translation block of CEBPA mRNA.[51,52] However, complete loss of CEBPA, experimentally performed by transducing BCR-ABL into primitive murine cells engineered to have CEPBA deleted, confers an erythroid leukemia rather than a myeloproliferative disease.[53] This implies that some residual CEPBA activity must be present, even in blast crisis, and that disturbances in proliferation in CML progression may result from subtle changes in the regulation of factors critical in controlling the flow of hematopoietic differentiation.

Genes associated with the maintenance of stem cell renewal have been logically associated with progression. Data from several sources seem to be converging on the Wnt/β-catenin pathway as critical for the evolution of CML. The Wnt/β-catenin signaling pathway has come front and center in normal and abnormal hematopoiesis. Wnt/β-catenin signaling is thought to be important in cell self-renewal, and mutations in β-catenin have been found in various epithelial solid tumors.[54–56] Aberrant Wnt/β-catenin signaling has thus been demonstrated in CML and T-lineage acute lymphoblastic leukemia (ALL).[57,58] In CML, activation of the Wnt/β-catenin pathway was observed in primary cell samples from patients with CML, with levels increasing with progression.[58] β-Catenin activation in CML seemed to reside predominately in granulocyte-macrophage progenitor cells, and the self-renewal of these progenitors could be reduced by overexpression of Axin, which modulates free β-catenin.

Several transcription factors appear to be involved in CML progression. Jun B knock-out mice develop a myeloproliferative disorder similar to CML.[6,59] Jun B has been shown to be downregulated in CML progression, and the decrease in junB does not appear to be mediated by methylation changes of junB promoters.[6,60] Genes controlled by the transcription factors MZF1 and delta EF1 appear to be deregulated in CML progression.[6,59] MZF1 is a member of the Kruppel family of zinc finger proteins originally cloned from a cDNA library from a blast-crisis CML patient,[61] and plays a critical role in hematopoietic stem cell differentiation, including modulation of CD34 and c-myb expression,[62,63] and MZF1$^{-/-}$ knock-out mice display an increase in hematopoietic progenitor proliferation, which continues in long-term culture conditions.[62] Both MZF1 and delta EF1 have been shown to influence cadherin expression.[64–66] Moreover, MDFI, an inhibitor of myogenic basic helix-loop-helix transcription factors found overexpressed in CML progression,[6] both interacts with axin and influences Jun signaling, thus perhaps linking these two pathways implicated in CML progression.[67,68]

WHERE DOES PROGRESSION OCCUR?

The primary lesion initiating CML likely takes place in a pluripotent stem cell, as the Ph can be encountered in myeloid and lymphoid lineages. Blast crisis involves the myeloid lineage in approximately 75% of cases while lymphoid blast crisis occurs in the remaining cases. (Curiously, lymphoid accelerated phase is never described, either because seeing any increase in lymphoid blasts triggers the diagnosis of lymphoid blast crisis, or because the disease kinetics are sufficiently fast as to make it difficult to catch in between chronic and blast phase.) For many years the natural assumption was that the primary changes in progression must take place at a fairly undifferentiated cell (perhaps a leukemia stem cell), thereby being able to proceed through myeloid or lymphoid lineages.

Several lines of evidence lead to a pause in this neat description. First came the landmark article by Jamieson and colleagues,[58] who studied the activation of β-catenin signaling in CML progression. These investigators found that the predominant changes in β-catenin activation occurred not in the immature Lin-CD34$^+$ 38- (LSC?) compartment, but in the Lin-CD34$^+$CD38$^+$ granulocyte-monocyte progenitor (GMP) fraction. It is not clear, however, whether the fundamental biological changes (mutations, gene expression, and so forth) were restricted to the GMP fraction, or if they occurred upstream in a more primitive cell, with subsequent unveiling of differential pathway activation (β-catenin) in the context of differentiation to the GMP compartment. However, some changes associated with progression appear to be lineage specific and, thus, probably occur at some point of differentiation from the LSC. Therefore, p53 and RUNX1 lesions occur predominately in myeloid blast crisis, whereas Ikaros transcription factor (IKZF1) and cyclin-dependent kinase inhibitor 2A/B changes occur in lymphoid blast crisis. (An alternative hypothesis is that these changes occur at the LSC level, but the changes are permissive to differentiation along only one of the myeloid or lymphoid pathways.)[48,49,69]

The involvement of IKZF1 in lymphoid blast crisis is an extension of studies of Ph+ ALL. Mullighan and colleagues[69] found an exceptionally high loss of the IKZF1 gene (coding for Ikaros) in Ph+ ALL cases. Of the 43 Ph+ cases studied, 36 (84%) had deletions in IKZF1. In 19 cases, the deletion was restricted to the region coding Ikaros exons 3 to 6 (designated the Ik6 variant). This isoform lacks the DNA binding domain while retaining the dimerization domains in exon 7, and acts as a dominant negative inhibitor of Ikaros that halts B-cell differentiation and contributes to the aberrant expression of some myeloid specific genes.[27] Chronic-phase CML was free of alterations in the IKZF1 site. Four of 15 blast-crisis samples showed an IKZF1 deletion, including 2/3 lymphoid blast crisis. Thus, though Ikaros involvement appears to be a predominately lymphoid event, it is rarely encountered in myeloid blast crisis.

HOW CAN WE TREAT PROGRESSION?

No treatment—be it interferon, TKI, or allogeneic transplantation—works well in advanced-phase disease. For example, even allogeneic transplant provides a long-term survival in only 25% to 40% of accelerated-phase patients and in about 10% of blast-crisis patients.[70] Why doesn't TKI cure blast-crisis patients? The initial response of blast-crisis patients suggest that blasts are overdependent on BCR-ABL–driven differentiation and apoptosis blockade; disruption of BCR-ABL thus provides "pharmaceutical judo" whereby cells stumble and pour through differentiation and death. However, the remaining LSC, presumably still primed with aberrant pathways, either develop new methods of BCR-ABL resistance or are free to proliferate using BCR-ABL–independent activation.

The biology of progression suggests that some therapies are aimed at moving primitive cells from self-renewal toward differentiation (targeting the Wnt/β-catenin and hedgehog pathways[71]) through inactivation of BCR-ABL signaling (PP2A activators[72]), targeting MAPK-driven proliferation and apoptosis (farnesyl transferase inhibitors,[73] demethylating agents), using antioxidants to prevent ROS damage,[74] and so forth (**Table 3**), although it is hard to imagine these regimens will have more "punch" than an allogeneic transplant, which leverages both cytotoxic and immunologic effects but still is woefully inadequate in blast-phase CML.

Any model of the pathogenesis and progression of CML must reconcile that (1) that response to therapy maps closely to phase of disease; (2) that response in blast phase is predictable but brief; and (3) that despite the stereotypic clinical progression of

Table 3
New drugs and pathways to target in CML?

Drug	Gene/Pathway	Comment
SMO inhibitors	Hedgehog/self-renewal	Various in trials
Forskolin, FTY720	PP2A	In trials
Hydroxychloroquine	Autophagy	Not yet in trials
Farnesyltransferase inhibitors; other MAPK inhibitors	MAPK activation/proliferation	Not yet in trials
Demethylating agents, histone deacetylase inhibitors	Multiple targeting aberrant gene expression	Various in trials

CML, the genetic lesions associated with progression are vast. **Fig. 1** is an attempt to model the process of progression. Early in the disease the Ph occurs in a primitive "stem cell" (process "y" in the figure), and BCR-ABL drives the process of chronic phase, spawning scores of leukemia progenitors (green clones). At this early juncture one must ask if the Ph is the first lesion in the leukemogenic process (x). First, the mere acquisition of the Ph suggests some genetic instability in a precursor causing the Ph. In addition, new clonal cytogenetic changes occur in more than 5% of chronic phases in CCyR, suggesting an ongoing genetic instability.[41,75,76] In addition, BCR-ABL has been found to occur in the peripheral blood of normal individuals (at a very low level) in an age-dependent manner, suggesting that the Ph may not be sufficient alone to cause leukemia. (But a caveat: these normal individuals have not been followed for long, and perhaps the Ph in these cases originated in a myeloid precursor, not a stem cell. If so, the Ph clone might be quite short-lived.)[77,78]

As the chronic phase continues without therapy, the genetic instability causes a change the clonal spectrum. If we imagine that the effects of genetic instability occur genome wide, it stands to reason that multiple genes will be affected. Some of these "hits" will be neutral (not affecting the fitness of the cell with the new mutation), other

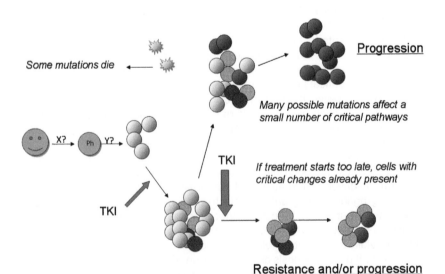

Some mutations die

Progression

Many possible mutations affect a small number of critical pathways

TKI

If treatment starts too late, cells with critical changes already present

TKI

Resistance and/or progression

Fig. 1. A simple model of CML progression/resistance.

mutations will be lethal to the affected cell, and still other mutations will offer a selective advantage. Thus, any gene in pathways that increases fitness—proliferation, cell renewal, apoptosis—have similar effects in promoting progression. This process may explain why there is a plethora of genes associated with progression.

Therefore the consequences of instability link resistance and progression. In **Fig. 1**, the bottom panel shows the expansion of chronic phase, with multiple clones occurring if TKI therapy is delayed. If TKI therapy is initiated early in the disease process (small red arrow), the disease is controlled. If the TKI therapy is delayed (large red arrow), critical changes are already present; indeed, the process has passed a "point of no return," and resistance and progression are likely. If some of the early changes involve genetic changes critical to progression, the process escalates (top panel) to progressive disease.

How to treat progression, then? It is likely that the only effective method to treat progression will be to prevent progression. There may be several ways to accomplish this mission. The first is stronger inhibition of BCR-ABL; this is the most compelling reason to use the stronger second-generation TKIs (dasatinib and nilotinib). However, in cases where there has been prolonged unopposed activity of BCR-ABL, a broader attack may be useful to further target the CML stem cell (assuming this exists). How does one tell which patients are far along the road to progression? Clinical features may suffice (the Sokal or Hansford score); alternatively, assays based on gene expression,[79] or the sensitive and early detection of Abl point mutations,[80] have great promise.

In the game of Clue, players must solve a mystery by tying together the assailant (eg, Professor Plum), the weapon (eg, the candlestick), and the location (eg, the library). Alas, biology is not a board game (or the author might be rich on Park Place, rather than writing academic reviews), so the culprit and crime are not so easy to deduce. Certainly BCR-ABL is the "brains" behind the pathogenesis and progression of CML, though along the way it recruits a bevy of accomplices that facilitate resistance and progression despite the prosecution of TKI, chemotherapy, and/or immunologic therapy. Advances in biological models (eg, murine) and technology (eg, gene expression arrays) have slowly shed some light onto the complexity of progression. It is hoped that the continued work to understand the progression program in CML will lead to successful innovations in diagnostics and therapeutics.

REFERENCES

1. Branford S, Rudzki Z, Walsh S, et al. Detection of BCR-ABL mutations in patients with CML treated with imatinib is virtually always accompanied by clinical resistance, and mutations in the ATP phosphate-binding loop (P-loop) are associated with a poor prognosis. Blood 2003;102(1):276–83.
2. Soverini S, Martinelli G, Rosti G, et al. ABL mutations in late chronic phase chronic myeloid leukemia patients with up-front cytogenetic resistance to imatinib are associated with a greater likelihood of progression to blast crisis and shorter survival: a study by the GIMEMA Working Party on Chronic Myeloid Leukemia. J Clin Oncol 2005;23(18):4100–9.
3. Melo JV, Barnes DJ. Chronic myeloid leukaemia as a model of disease evolution in human cancer. Nat Rev Cancer 2007;7(6):441–53.
4. Perrotti D, Jamieson C, Goldman J, et al. Chronic myeloid leukemia: mechanisms of blastic transformation. J Clin Invest 2010;120(7):2254–64.
5. O'Brien S, Berman E, Bhalla K, et al. Chronic myelogenous leukemia. J Natl Compr Canc Netw 2007;5(5):474–96.

6. Radich JP, Dai H, Mao M, et al. Gene expression changes associated with progression and response in chronic myeloid leukemia. Proc Natl Acad Sci U S A 2006;103(8):2794–9.

7. Au WY, Caguioa PB, Chuah C, et al. Chronic myeloid leukemia in Asia. Int J Hematol 2009;89(1):14–23.

8. Branford S, Rudzki Z, Walsh S, et al. High frequency of point mutations clustered within the adenosine triphosphate-binding region of BCR/ABL in patients with chronic myeloid leukemia or Ph-positive acute lymphoblastic leukemia who develop imatinib (STI571) resistance. Blood 2002;99(9):3472–5.

9. Branford S, Rudzki Z, Harper A, et al. Imatinib produces significantly superior molecular responses compared to interferon alfa plus cytarabine in patients with newly diagnosed chronic myeloid leukemia in chronic phase. Leukemia 2003;17(12):2401–9.

10. Shah NP, Nicoll JM, Nagar B, et al. Multiple BCR-ABL kinase domain mutations confer polyclonal resistance to the tyrosine kinase inhibitor imatinib (STI571) in chronic phase and blast crisis chronic myeloid leukemia. Cancer Cell 2002;2(2):117–25.

11. Koptyra M, Falinski R, Nowickl MO, et al. BCR/ABL kinase induces self-mutagenesis via reactive oxygen species to encode imatinib resistance. Blood 2006;108(1):319–27.

12. Chu S, Xu H, Shah NP, et al. Detection of BCR-ABL kinase mutations in CD34+ cells from chronic myelogenous leukemia patients in complete cytogenetic remission on imatinib mesylate treatment. Blood 2005;105(5):2093–8.

13. Jiang X, Saw KM, Eaves A, et al. Instability of BCR-ABL gene in primary and cultured chronic myeloid leukemia stem cells. J Natl Cancer Inst 2007;99(9):680–93.

14. Collins SJ, Groudine MT. Chronic myelogenous leukemia: amplification of a rearranged c-abl oncogene in both chronic phase and blast crisis. Blood 1987;69(3):893–8.

15. Huntly BJ, Bench AJ, Delabesse E, et al. Derivative chromosome 9 deletions in chronic myeloid leukemia: poor prognosis is not associated with loss of ABL-BCR expression, elevated BCR-ABL levels, or karyotypic instability. Blood 2002;99(12):4547–53.

16. Huntly BJ, Guilhot F, Reid AG, et al. Imatinib improves but may not fully reverse the poor prognosis of patients with CML with derivative chromosome 9 deletions. Blood 2003;102(6):2205–12.

17. Sawyers CL, McLaughlin J, Witte ON. Genetic requirement for Ras in the transformation of fibroblasts and hematopoietic cells by the Bcr-Abl oncogene. J Exp Med 1995;181(1):307–13.

18. Ilaria RL Jr, Van Etten RA. P210 and P190(BCR/ABL) induce the tyrosine phosphorylation and DNA binding activity of multiple specific STAT family members. J Biol Chem 1996;271(49):31704–10.

19. Shuai K, Halpern J, ten Hoeve J, et al. Constitutive activation of STAT5 by the BCR-ABL oncogene in chronic myelogenous leukemia. Oncogene 1996;13(2):247–54.

20. Skorski T, Kanakaraj P, Nieborowska-Skorska M, et al. Phosphatidylinositol-3 kinase activity is regulated by BCR/ABL and is required for the growth of Philadelphia chromosome-positive cells. Blood 1995;86(2):726–36.

21. Salgia R, Uemura N, Okuda K, et al. CRKL links p210BCR/ABL with paxillin in chronic myelogenous leukemia cells. J Biol Chem 1995;270(49):29145–50.

22. Barnes DJ, Palaiologou D, Panousopoulou E, et al. Bcr-Abl expression levels determine the rate of development of resistance to imatinib mesylate in chronic myeloid leukemia. Cancer Res 2005;65(19):8912–9.

23. Barnes DJ, Schultheis B, Adedeji S, et al. Dose-dependent effects of Bcr-Abl in cell line models of different stages of chronic myeloid leukemia. Oncogene 2005;24(42):6432–40.

24. Modi H, McDonald T, Chu S, et al. Role of BCR/ABL gene-expression levels in determining the phenotype and imatinib sensitivity of transformed human hematopoietic cells. Blood 2007;109(12):5411–21.

25. Perrotti D, Neviani P. From mRNA metabolism to cancer therapy: chronic myelogenous leukemia shows the way. Clin Cancer Res 2007;13(6):1638–42.

26. Abrahamsson AE, Geron I, Gotlib J, et al. Glycogen synthase kinase 3beta missplicing contributes to leukemia stem cell generation. Proc Natl Acad Sci U S A 2009;106(10):3925–9.

27. Klein F, Feldhahn N, Herzog S, et al. BCR-ABL1 induces aberrant splicing of IKAROS and lineage infidelity in pre-B lymphoblastic leukemia cells. Oncogene 2006;25(7):1118–24.

28. Yu J, Vodyanik MA, Smuga-Otto K, et al. Induced pluripotent stem cell lines derived from human somatic cells. Science 2007;318(5858):1917–20.

29. Viswanathan SR, Powers JT, Einhorn W, et al. Lin28 promotes transformation and is associated with advanced human malignancies. Nat Genet 2009;41(7):843–8.

30. Calabretta B, Perrotti D. The biology of CML blast crisis. Blood 2004;103(11): 4010–22.

31. Shet AS, Jahagirdar BN, Verfaillie CM. Chronic myelogenous leukemia: mechanisms underlying disease progression. Leukemia 2002;16(8):1402–11.

32. Skorski T. Oncogenic tyrosine kinases and the DNA-damage response. Nat Rev Cancer 2002;2(5):351–60.

33. Majsterek I, Blasiak J, Mlynarski W, et al. Does the BCR/ABL-mediated increase in the efficacy of DNA repair play a role in the drug resistance of cancer cells? Cell Biol Int 2002;26(4):363–70.

34. Slupianek A, Hoser G, Majsterek I, et al. Fusion tyrosine kinases induce drug resistance by stimulation of homology-dependent recombination repair, prolongation of G(2)/M phase, and protection from apoptosis. Mol Cell Biol 2002; 22(12):4189–201.

35. Sattler M, Verma S, Shrikhande G, et al. The BCR/ABL tyrosine kinase induces production of reactive oxygen species in hematopoietic cells. J Biol Chem 2000;275(32):24273–8.

36. Fioretos T, Strombeck B, Sandberg T, et al. Isochromosome 17q in blast crisis of chronic myeloid leukemia and in other hematologic malignancies is the result of clustered breakpoints in 17p11 and is not associated with coding TP53 mutations. Blood 1999;94(1):225–32.

37. Levine AJ. p53, the cellular gatekeeper for growth and division. Cell 1997;88(3): 323–31.

38. Sawyers CL, Callahan W, Witte ON. Dominant negative MYC blocks transformation by ABL oncogenes. Cell 1992;70(6):901–10.

39. Collins S, Groudine M. Amplification of endogenous myc-related DNA sequences in a human myeloid leukaemia cell line. Nature 1982;298(5875):679–81.

40. Virtaneva K, Wright FA, Tanner SM, et al. Expression profiling reveals fundamental biological differences in acute myeloid leukemia with isolated trisomy 8 and normal cytogenetics. Proc Natl Acad Sci U S A 2001;98(3):1124–9.

41. Medina J, Kantarjian H, Talpaz M, et al. Chromosomal abnormalities in Philadelphia chromosome-negative metaphases appearing during imatinib mesylate therapy in patients with Philadelphia chromosome-positive chronic myelogenous leukemia in chronic phase. Cancer 2003;98(9):1905–11.

42. Mitani K, Ogawa S, Tanaka T, et al. Generation of the AML1-EVI-1 fusion gene in the t(3;21)(q26;q22) causes blastic crisis in chronic myelocytic leukemia. EMBO J 1994;13(3):504–10.

43. Nakamura T, Largaespada DA, Lee MP, et al. Fusion of the nucleoporin gene NUP98 to HOXA9 by the chromosome translocation t(7;11)(p15;p15) in human myeloid leukaemia. Nat Genet 1996;12(2):154–8.

44. Cuenco GM, Ren R. Cooperation of BCR-ABL and AML1/MDS1/EVI1 in blocking myeloid differentiation and rapid induction of an acute myelogenous leukemia. Oncogene 2001;20(57):8236–48.

45. Dash AB, Williams IR, Kutok JL, et al. A murine model of CML blast crisis induced by cooperation between BCR/ABL and NUP98/HOXA9. Proc Natl Acad Sci U S A 2002;99(11):7622–7.

46. Ito T, Kwon HY, Zimdahl B, et al. Regulation of myeloid leukaemia by the cell-fate determinant Musashi. Nature 2010;466(7307):765–8.

47. Collins SJ, Howard M, Andrews DF, et al. Rare occurrence of N-ras point mutations in Philadelphia chromosome positive chronic myeloid leukemia. Blood 1989;73(4):1028–32.

48. Ahuja H, Bar-Eli M, Advani SH, et al. Alterations in the p53 gene and the clonal evolution of the blast crisis of chronic myelocytic leukemia. Proc Natl Acad Sci U S A 1989;86(17):6783–7.

49. Sill H, Goldman JM, Cross NC. Homozygous deletions of the p16 tumor-suppressor gene are associated with lymphoid transformation of chronic myeloid leukemia. Blood 1995;85(8):2013–6.

50. Neviani P, Santhanam R, Trotta R, et al. The tumor suppressor PP2A is functionally inactivated in blast crisis CML through the inhibitory activity of the BCR/ABL-regulated SET protein. Cancer Cell 2005;8(5):355–68.

51. Chang JS, Santhanam R, Trotta R, et al. High levels of the BCR/ABL oncoprotein are required for the MAPK-hnRNP-E2 dependent suppression of C/EBPalpha-driven myeloid differentiation. Blood 2007;110(3):994–1003.

52. Perrotti D, Cesi V, Trotta R, et al. BCR-ABL suppresses C/EBPalpha expression through inhibitory action of hnRNP E2. Nat Genet 2002;30(1):48–58.

53. Wagner K, Zhang P, Rosenbauer F, et al. Absence of the transcription factor CCAAT enhancer binding protein alpha results in loss of myeloid identity in bcr/abl-induced malignancy. Proc Natl Acad Sci U S A 2006;103(16):6338–43.

54. Korinek V, Barker N, Morin PJ, et al. Constitutive transcriptional activation by a beta-catenin-Tcf complex in APC-/- colon carcinoma. Science 1997;275(5307):1784–7.

55. Rask K, Nilsson A, Brannstrom M, et al. Wnt-signalling pathway in ovarian epithelial tumours: increased expression of beta-catenin and GSK3beta. Br J Cancer 2003;89(7):1298–304.

56. Uematsu K, He B, You L, et al. Activation of the Wnt pathway in non small cell lung cancer: evidence of dishevelled overexpression. Oncogene 2003;22(46):7218–21.

57. Guo Z, Dose M, Kovalovsky D, et al. {beta}-Catenin stabilization stalls the transition from double-positive to single-positive stage and predisposes thymocytes to malignant transformation. Blood 2007;109(12):5463–72.

58. Jamieson CH, Ailles LE, Dylla SJ, et al. Granulocyte-macrophage progenitors as candidate leukemic stem cells in blast-crisis CML. N Engl J Med 2004;351(7):657–67.

59. Passegue E, Wagner EF, Weissman IL. JunB deficiency leads to a myeloproliferative disorder arising from hematopoietic stem cells. Cell 2004;119(3):431–43.

60. Hoshino K, Quintas-Cardama A, Radich J, et al. Downregulation of JUNB mRNA expression in advanced phase chronic myelogenous leukemia. Leuk Res 2009; 33(10):1361–6.
61. Hromas R, Collins SJ, Hickstein D, et al. A retinoic acid-responsive human zinc finger gene, MZF-1, preferentially expressed in myeloid cells. J Biol Chem 1991;266(22):14183–7.
62. Gaboli M, Kotsi PA, Gurrieri C, et al. Mzf1 controls cell proliferation and tumorigenesis. Genes Dev 2001;15(13):1625–30.
63. Perrotti D, Melotti P, Skorski T, et al. Overexpression of the zinc finger protein MZF1 inhibits hematopoietic development from embryonic stem cells: correlation with negative regulation of CD34 and c-myb promoter activity. Mol Cell Biol 1995; 15(11):6075–87.
64. Guaita S, Puig I, Franci C, et al. Snail induction of epithelial to mesenchymal transition in tumor cells is accompanied by MUC1 repression and ZEB1 expression. J Biol Chem 2002;277(42):39209–16.
65. Le Mee S, Fromigue O, Marie PJ. Sp1/Sp3 and the myeloid zinc finger gene MZF1 regulate the human N-cadherin promoter in osteoblasts. Exp Cell Res 2005;302(1):129–42.
66. Miyoshi A, Kitajima Y, Sumi K, et al. Snail and SIP1 increase cancer invasion by upregulating MMP family in hepatocellular carcinoma cells. Br J Cancer 2004; 90(6):1265–73.
67. Kusano S, Raab-Traub N. I-Mfa domain proteins interact with Axin and affect its regulation of the Wnt and c-Jun N-terminal kinase signaling pathways. Mol Cell Biol 2002;22(18):6393–405.
68. Nelson WJ, Nusse R. Convergence of Wnt, beta-catenin, and cadherin pathways. Science 2004;303(5663):1483–7.
69. Mullighan CG, Miller CB, Radtke I, et al. BCR-ABL1 lymphoblastic leukaemia is characterized by the deletion of Ikaros. Nature 2008;453(7191):110–4.
70. Gratwohl A, Stern M, Brand R, et al. Risk score for outcome after allogeneic hematopoietic stem cell transplantation: a retrospective analysis. Cancer 2009; 115(20):4715–26.
71. Zhao C, Chen A, Jamieson CH, et al. Hedgehog signalling is essential for maintenance of cancer stem cells in myeloid leukaemia. Nature 2009;458(7239): 776–9.
72. Perrotti D, Neviani P. Protein phosphatase 2A (PP2A), a drugable tumor suppressor in Ph1(+) leukemias. Cancer Metastasis Rev 2008;27(2):159–68.
73. Copland M, Pellicano F, Richmond L, et al. BMS-214662 potently induces apoptosis of chronic myeloid leukemia stem and progenitor cells and synergizes with tyrosine kinase inhibitors. Blood 2008;111(5):2843–53.
74. Skorski T. BCR/ABL, DNA damage and DNA repair: implications for new treatment concepts. Leuk Lymphoma 2008;49(4):610–4.
75. Bumm T, Muller C, Al-Ali HK, et al. Emergence of clonal cytogenetic abnormalities in Ph- cells in some CML patients in cytogenetic remission to imatinib but restoration of polyclonal hematopoiesis in the majority. Blood 2003;101(5):1941–9.
76. O'Dwyer ME, Gatter KM, Loriaux M, et al. Demonstration of Philadelphia chromosome negative abnormal clones in patients with chronic myelogenous leukemia during major cytogenetic responses induced by imatinib mesylate. Leukemia 2003;17(3):481–7.
77. Biernaux C, Loos M, Sels A, et al. Detection of major bcr-abl gene expression at a very low level in blood cells of some healthy individuals. Blood 1995;86(8): 3118–22.

78. Bose S, Deininger M, Gora-Tybor J, et al. The presence of typical and atypical BCR-ABL fusion genes in leukocytes of normal individuals: biologic significance and implications for the assessment of minimal residual disease. Blood 1998; 92(9):3362–7.
79. Oehler VG, Yeung KY, Choi YE, et al. The derivation of diagnostic markers of chronic myeloid leukemia progression from microarray data. Blood 2009; 114(15):3292–8.
80. Oehler VG, Qin J, Ramakrishnan R, et al. Absolute quantitative detection of ABL tyrosine kinase domain point mutations in chronic myeloid leukemia using a novel nanofluidic platform and mutation-specific PCR. Leukemia 2009;23(2):396–9.

Chronic Myeloid Leukemia: Mechanisms of Resistance and Treatment

Elias Jabbour, MD*, Sameer A. Parikh, MD, Hagop Kantarjian, MD,
Jorge Cortes, MD

KEYWORDS

- Myeloproliferative disorders • Tyrosine kinase inhibitors
- Mutation screening • Homoharringtonine
- Multikinase inhibitors

Chronic myeloid leukemia (CML) is a pluripotent hematopoietic stem cell disorder leading to myeloproliferation and its attendant consequences. In the United States, it is estimated that approximately 5050 cases of CML will be diagnosed in 2010 with an annual incidence of 1 to 2 cases per 100,000 adults.[1] The instigating factor in the pathogenesis of CML is the formation of the Philadelphia chromosome resulting from the reciprocal translocation between chromosomes 9 and 22 (t[9;22][q34;q11]), which is associated with the de novo creation of the *BCR-ABL* fusion oncogene.[2,3] The gene product of the *BCR-ABL* gene constitutively activates numerous downstream targets including *c-myc*, *Akt*, and *Jun*, all of which cause uncontrolled proliferation and survival of CML cells.

IMATINIB MESYLATE

Imatinib mesylate (Gleevec, STI-571), a 2-phenylaminopyrimidine, is a selective and potent inhibitor of *BCR-ABL* and a few other tyrosine kinases, including *c-kit*, *PDGF-R* α and β, and *ABL*-related gene.[4] It is orally administered with 98% bioavailability and a half-life of 13 to 16 hours. Imatinib was first used in patients with CML who had developed resistance or intolerance to interferon (IFN)-α. Among 532 such patients treated with imatinib, a complete cytogenetic response (CCyR) was achieved in 60%. The estimated 5-year survival rate was 76%.[5,6]

Based on these favorable results, a large, randomized trial was initiated among patients with CML in chronic phase (CML-CP) who had received no prior therapy. In

The University of Texas MD Anderson Cancer Center, Houston, TX, USA
* Corresponding author. Department of Leukemia, The University of Texas MD Anderson Cancer Center, Box 428, 1515 Holcombe Boulevard, Houston, TX 77030.
E-mail address: ejabbour@mdanderson.org

Hematol Oncol Clin N Am 25 (2011) 981–995
doi:10.1016/j.hoc.2011.09.004
0889-8588/11/$ – see front matter © 2011 Elsevier Inc. All rights reserved.

this study, known as the International Randomized Study of Interfreron versus STI571 (IRIS) trial, patients were randomized to receive imatinib or IFN-α and ara-C, which was the standard therapy at the time. Treatment with imatinib was significantly better in nearly all outcomes measured, including hematologic and cytogenetic response, toxicity, and progression-free survival (PFS).[7] After 8 years, the cumulative CCyR rate for first-line imatinib-treated patients was 82%.[8] The event-free survival (EFS) was 81%, and the estimated rate of freedom from progression to accelerated phase (CML-AP) or blastic phase (CML-BP) was 92%. The estimated overall survival (OS) rate for patients treated with imatinib was 85%. At 8 years, 304 patients (55%) randomized to imatinib remained on treatment. The curves seem to plateau after the fourth year and yearly event rates have ranged from 0.3% to 2%. With an annual mortality of 2%, the estimated survival of a newly diagnosed patient with CML may be in the range of 20 to 30 years.

Mechanisms of Resistance

Despite the impressive results with imatinib, a subset of patients treated with imatinib develops resistance. Failure to achieve a landmark response is considered primary resistance, and this is further subdivided into primary hematologic resistance and primary cytogenetic resistance. Secondary resistance is defined by the achievement and then subsequent loss of a hematologic or cytogenetic response. Hematologic resistance occurs in 2% to 4% of cases, whereas cytogenetic resistance is more common, occurring in 15% to 25% of patients. Mutations in BCR-ABL are rarely responsible for primary resistance. Recent work suggests that primary resistance may be associated with increased transcript levels of the drug metabolism gene prostaglandin–endoperoxide synthase 1/cyclooxgenase 1, and this may serve as a biomarker to distinguish patients with primary resistance to imatinib.[9]

Several mechanisms of resistance to imatinib have been described. These can be classified into two categories: BCR-ABL–dependent and BCR-ABL–independent. The first group includes amplification or overexpression of BCR-ABL or its protein product,[10] and point mutations of the ABL sequence.[11] The second group includes multidrug-resistance expression and overexpression of Src kinases.[12] BCR-ABL–dependent mechanisms are more common, particularly point mutations, which have been identified in approximately 50% of patients who develop clinical resistance to imatinib.[13,14] More than 90 different mutations have been described and occur in any of the different relevant domains of the kinase, including the ATP-binding domain (also known as P-loop), the catalytic domain, the activation loop, and amino acids that make direct contact with imatinib. The significance of these mutations varies. Although some retain some sensitivity to imatinib at concentrations similar to those of the wild-type sequence others, particularly T315I, are nearly completely insensitive to imatinib.[15] Most of the clinically relevant mutations develop in a few residues in the in the P-loop (G250E, Y253F/H, and E255K/V); the contact site (T315I); and the catalytic domain (M351T and F359V).[16] The P-loop mutations have been suggested to carry an increased risk of rapid blastic transformation and short survival,[13] although the MD Anderson Cancer Center (MDACC) experience does not support this notion.[17] In some patients, more than one mutation may be present at the same time. This phenomenon seems to increase in frequency after treatment with more than one tyrosine kinase mutation. Mutations are quantified by direct sequencing and the sensitivity of such assay varies between 10% and 25%.[18,19] Other methods, such as denatured high-performance liquid chromatography, increase the sensitivity to 1% to 10%.[19,20] However, it is unclear at this time if identification of small mutated clones with these highly sensitive methods is clinically relevant.

Other mechanisms of resistance caused by intrinsic factors include *BCR-ABL* gene amplification, *BCR-ABL* overexpression, aberrations in other oncogenetic signaling pathways, and the persistence of leukemic stem cells.[14,21,22] Extrinsic factors contributing to resistance include those that decrease the blood levels or bioavailability of imatinib, such as patient compliance, drug–drug interactions, drug influx and efflux, and multidrug resistance in sanctuary sites, and microenvironmental factors.[21]

Mutation Screening During Imatinib Therapy

The European LeukemiaNet (ELN) and the National Comprehensive Cancer Network provide guidance for the monitoring of patients with CML.[23,24] The criteria for defining optimal response, suboptimal response, and failure to respond are outlined in **Table 1**. The ELN recommends mutational analysis in instances of suboptimal response or failure to therapy, and always before changing therapy to a second-generation tyrosine kinase inhibitor (TKI). Patients failing TKI therapy should potentially be assessed for compliance to therapy before switch, because it has been shown that patient-reported compliance and actual compliance reported can be discordant, and this may be a reason for treatment failure. The magnitude of increase in *BCR-ABL* transcript levels that should prompt mutation testing is a topic of debate. Fivefold to 10-fold rises have been proposed as a reasonable trigger for mutation testing. A recent study demonstrated that increases in *BCR-ABL* mRNA levels of fivefold or more were not sufficiently sensitive in detecting mutations, and that a 2.6-fold increase in *BCR-ABL* transcripts is a better threshold.[25] In most clinics, however, it may be more reasonable to consider mutation testing when *BCR-ABL* levels increase at least fivefold, confirmed in an independent test in the same laboratory to confirm that the observed increase is real, and not caused by assay or laboratory variability.

Strategies to Overcome Imatinib Resistance

Multiple strategies to overcome failure to standard dose (400 mg/day) imatinib are under investigation. These include dose escalation of imatinib, switch to a second-generation TKI, other novel TKIs in a clinical trial, non–TKI-based therapy, and allogeneic stem cell transplant in eligible patients.

Imatinib Dose Escalation

Dose escalation can improve the response in a subset of patients with resistance to standard-dose imatinib and was the main option for managing suboptimal responses

Table 1
Response definitions to imatinib in chronic phase CML (European Leukemia Net guidelines)

Evaluation Time	Response		
	Optimal	Suboptimal	Failure
3 months	CHR and at least minor CyR	No CyR	No CHR
6 months	At least partial CyR	Less than partial CyR	No CyR
12 months	CCyR	Partial CyR	Less than partial CyR
18 months	MMR	Less than MMR	Less than CCyR
Any time	Stable or improving MMR	Loss of MMR, presence of mutations	Loss of CHR, loss of CCyR, clonal evolution

Abbreviations: CCyR, complete cytogenetic response; CHR, complete hematologic response; CyR, cytogenetic response; MMR, major molecular response.

and treatment failures before the introduction of second-generation TKIs. In a retrospective analysis of patients enrolled in the IRIS trial, Kantarjian and colleagues[26] reported that among 106 patients who required dose escalation because of resistance to standard-dose therapy, freedom-from-progression and OS rates were 89% and 84%, respectively, at 3 years from dose escalation. In another study from MDACC, 84 patients with CML-CP were dose escalated to imatinib, 600 to 800 mg/day, after developing hematologic failure (n = 21) or cytogenetic failure (n = 63) to standard-dose imatinib.[27] Among patients who met the criteria for cytogenetic failure, 75% (47 of 63) responded to imatinib dose escalation. In contrast, in patients where imatinib was dose escalated because of hematologic failure, 48% achieved a complete hematologic response (CHR) and only 14% (3 of 21) achieved a cytogenetic response. Patients more likely to respond to imatinib dose increase are those who have previously achieved a cytogenetic response and then lost it and who have not developed any mutations unresponsive to imatinib. Even in these cases, a switch to a second-generation TKI is preferable unless the patient has no access to these agents.

Several Phase II studies examined the role of a higher dose of imatinib (800 mg) upfront in the treatment of patients with CML. The Tyrosine Kinase Inhibitor Optimization and Selectivity (TOPS) study was a Phase 3 trial comparing the efficacy and safety of high-dose (800 mg/day) with standard-dose imatinib (400 mg/day) in patients with newly diagnosed CML-CP.[28] The primary endpoint of the study was rate of major molecular response (MMR) at 12 months of therapy. A 24-month update on the TOPS data was recently reported.[29] It seems that there was no significant difference between the 800 and 400 mg/day arms for either the CCyR (76% vs 76%, respectively; P = 1.00) or MMR rate (51% vs 54%, respectively; P = .626). Most importantly, thus far at 24 months there were no differences between arms with respect to EFS (95% vs 95%, respectively; P = .71), PFS (98% vs 97%; P = .64), and OS (98% vs 97%, respectively; P = .70), although it is still relatively early. Adverse events tended to be more common among patients in the 800 mg/day arm versus the 400 mg/day arm, as was the rate of discontinuation caused by adverse events (12% vs 5%, respectively). The results from the TOPS study were confirmed in a randomized trial Gruppo Italiano Malattie Ematologiche dell'Adulto 021/ELN assessing the efficacy of imatinib 800 versus 400 mg/day as front-line therapy in high-risk Sokal patients.[30] The primary study endpoint of CCyR at 1 year was not significantly different between patients treated with imatinib 400 (61%) versus 800 mg/day (64%). There was a trend toward higher rates of MMR with 800 compared with 400 mg/day, but the differences were not statistically significant. Adverse events were not significantly different between treatment arms, but compliance was lower in the 800-mg arm (62% received doses >600 mg) compared with the 400-mg arm (87% received doses >350 mg).

Although the aforementioned studies have shown improved CCyR and MMR with a higher dose of imatinib, the follow-up of these studies is short to evaluate for EFS and OS. Hence, at the writing of this article, imatinib at a dose of 400 mg daily is still the preferred regimen of choice in patients newly diagnosed with CML-CP.

DASATINIB

Dasatinib (Sprycel; Bristol-Myers Squib, Princeton, NJ) is an orally bioavailable, multikinase inhibitor that is 325-fold more potent than imatinib against unmutated BCR-ABL.[31] It is currently approved for the treatment of imatinib-resistant or imatininb-intolerant CML in all phases and Ph-positive acute lymphoblastic leukemia. The response to dasatinib among patients in chronic, accelerated and blast phase (myeloid and lymphoid) after imatinib failure is summarized in **Table 2**.[32–34] Dasatinib

Table 2

Response to second-generation tyrosine kinase inhibitors (dasatinib, nilotinib, and bosutinib) in patients who are imatinib-resistant or -intolerant in chronic phase, accelerated phase, and blast phase CML

| | Percent Response | | | | | | | | | | |
| | Dasatinib | | | | Nilotinib | | | | Bosutinib | | |
Response	CP N = 387	AP N = 174	MyBP N = 109	LyBP N = 48	CP N = 321	AP N = 137	MyBP N = 105	LyBP N = 31	CP N = 146	AP N = 51	BP N = 38
Median follow-up (mo)	15	14	12+	12+	24	9	3	3	7	6	3
% Resistant to imatinib	74	93	91	88	70	80	82	82	69	NR	NR
% Hematologic response	—	79	50	40	94	56	22	19	85	54	36
CHR	91	45	27	29	76	31	11	13	81	54	36
NEL	—	19	7	6	—	12	1	0	—	0	0
% Cytogenetic response	NR	44	36	52	NR	NR	NR	NR	—	NR	NR
Complete	49	32	26	46	46	20	29	32	34	27	35
Partial	11	7	7	6	15	12	10	16	13	20	18
% Survival (at 12 mo)	96 (15)	82 (12)	50 (12)	50 (5)	87 (24)	67 (24)	42 (12)	42 (12)	98 (12)	60 (12)	50 (10)

Abbreviations: AP, accelerated phase; CHR, complete hematologic response; CP, chronic phase; LyBP, lymphoid blast phase; MyBP, myeloid blast phase; NEL, no evidence of leukemia.

is overall well tolerated. Myelosuppression occurs frequently, with grade 3 or 4 neutropenia or thrombocytopenia occurring in nearly 50% of patients treated at a dose of 70 mg twice daily (BID). The most common nonhematologic grade 3 to 4 toxicities at a dose of 70 mg BID were pleural effusion (9%); dyspnea (6%); bleeding (4%); diarrhea (3%); and fatigue (3%). In an open-label Phase III trial, 670 patients with imatinib-resistant and -intolerant CML-CP were randomly assigned among four dasatinib treatment schedules: (1) 100 mg once daily, (2) 50 mg BID, (3) 140 mg once daily, or (4) 70 mg BID.[35] Results of this trial showed that 100 mg once daily retained its activity and was associated with less toxicity, particularly pleural effusion and myelosuppression, with grade 3 to 4 neutropenia or thrombocytopenia occurring in approximately 30% each.

Based on these results, a Phase II trial from MDACC was recently reported in 50 patients with newly diagnosed chronic-phase CML.[36] Ninety-eight percent achieved CCyR and 41 patients (82%) achieved MMR. Responses occurred rapidly, with 94% of patients achieving CCyR by 6 months. The projected EFS rate at 24 months was 88%. A randomized Phase 3 trial comparing the efficacy of dasatinib and imatinib in the first-line has completed accrual, and results are expected in late 2010.

NILOTINIB

Nilotinib (Tasigna; Novartis Pharmaceuticals, East Hanover, NJ) is a rationally designed BCR-ABL inhibitor that is 30-fold more potent than imatinib in vitro, with greater specificity for BCR-ABL.[37,38] It is currently approved for treatment of imatinib-resistant and -intolerant patients with CML-CP and CML-AP (but not BP or Ph-positive acute lymphoblastic leukemia) at a dose of 400 mg BID. The response to nilotinib among patients in chronic, accelerated, and blast phase (myeloid and lymphoid) after imatinib failure is summarized in **Table 2**.[39,40] The most common grade 3 or 4 laboratory abnormalities were elevated lipase (17%); hypophosphatemia (16%); hyperglycemia (12%); and elevated total bilirubin (8%). Grade 3 or 4 nonhematologic adverse events were infrequent, with rash, headache, and diarrhea occurring in 2% of patients. The most common grade 3 or 4 hematologic adverse events were neutropenia (31%); thrombocytopenia (31%); and anemia (10%). Pleural or pericardial effusions (all grades) occurred in 2% of patients, and grade 3 or 4 pleural or pericardial effusions were rare (<1%).

Nilotinib has also demonstrated promise as a front-line therapy in patients with CML-CP.[41–43] In the first head-to-head comparison of a second-generation TKI (nilotinib at 300 or 400 mg BID) with imatinib (400 mg/day), nilotinib 300 and 400 mg BID showed higher rates of MMR (44% and 43%, respectively) and CCyR (80% and 78%, respectively) than imatinib at 400 mg/day (MMR, 22% [P<.0001 vs both nilotinib doses]; CCyR, 65% [P<.0001 vs nilotinib 300 mg BID; P<.0005 vs nilotinib 400 mg BID) at 12 months of follow-up.[42] In a Phase II study from MDACC, 51 patients with newly diagnosed CML-CP were treated with nilotinib at 400 mg BID. Ninety-eight percent of patients achieved CCyR, whereas 76% (39 of 51) achieved MMR. Rapid responses were observed, with 96% and 98% of patients in CCyR by 3 and 6 months, respectively.[41] A randomized Phase 3 trial comparing the efficacy of nilotinib and imatinib in the first-line has completed accrual, and results are expected in late 2010.

BOSUTINIB

Bosutinib (SKI606), an orally available dual SRC/ABL inhibitor, is 30 to 50 times more potent than imatinib, with minimal inhibitory activity against C-Kit and PDGFR, and expected to produce less myelosuppression and fluid retention.[44] The Phase I study identified a treatment dose of 500 mg daily and showed evidence of clinical efficacy. Phase II studies in patients with CML-CP who have failed imatinib and second-generation TKIs therapy are ongoing.[45,46] Preliminary data for response to nilotinib among patients in chronic, accelerated, and blast phase (myeloid and lymphoid) after imatinib failure are summarized in **Table 2**. The most common adverse events with bosutinib were gastrointestinal (nausea, vomiting, and diarrhea); these were usually grade 1 to 2, manageable and transient, and diminishing in frequency and severity after the first 3 to 4 weeks of treatment. Bosutinib is currently being assessed in the frontline setting for treatment of patients with CML-CP.

OTHER MULTIKINASE INHIBITORS

One of the most promising agents for treatment of T315I mutation in clinical trials is AP24534, an orally available multi-TKI designed using a structure-based approach as a pan–*BCR-ABL* inhibitor.[47] AP24534 potently inhibits the enzymatic activity of *BCR-ABL*-T315I, the native enzyme, and all other tested mutants. It also prevents the emergence of resistant mutants at concentrations of 40 nM. In a Phase 1 clinical trial of AP24534 at doses from 2 to 60 mg in 27 patients with CML (19 with CP, 4 AP, and 4 BP), CHR was achieved or maintained in 83% of patients treated in CP; major hematologic responses were also achieved in 38% of patients treated in advanced stages of the disease.[48] More importantly, 9 of 20 patients treated in CP achieved major cytogenetic response (including five CCyR), including three of seven with T315I (two CCyR). The most common drug-related adverse events were elevations of lipase and amylase at a dose of 60 mg daily. Grade 3 or 4 thrombocytopenia occurred in 9% of patients, with no grade 3 to 4 drug-related neutropenia. AP24534 will be tested in a large, multicenter study focusing on patients with imatinib-, niloti-nib-, and dasatinib-resistant disease, including a subset with the T315I mutation.

XL228 (Exelixis, San Francisco, CA) is a potent, multitargeted kinase inhibitor with potent activity against wild-type and T315I isoforms of *BCR-ABL*.[49] In a preliminary Phase 1 clinical study, XL228 was administered to 27 patients in six cohorts with a once-weekly dosing schedule (dose range, 0.45–10.8 mg/kg). All patients were resistant or intolerant to at least two prior standard therapies (including imatinib, dasa-tinib, and nilotinib) or had a known *BCR-ABL* T315I mutation. Preliminary evidence of clinical activity was observed in patients treated at doses of 3.6 mg/kg and higher, including stable or decreasing white blood cell or platelet count within 2 months (in 14 patients, 5 with T315I), or greater than 1-log reduction in *BCR-ABL* transcript levels by reverse-transcriptase polymerase chain reaction within 3 months (in three patients, two with T315I). XL 228 has been generally well tolerated. Dose-limiting toxicities observed with once-weekly dosing included grade 3 syncope and hyperglycemia in two patients dosed at 10.8 mg/kg. The most commonly reported grade 2 adverse effects were hyperglycemia, fatigue, nausea, vomiting, and bradycardia.

NON–TKIs

Homoharringtonine is a plant alkaloid that has been used in China for many years in the treatment of patients with acute myeloid leukemia. Before the introduction of ima-tinib, it was the best treatment option for patients who failed IFN-α and were not trans-plant candidates, with cytogenetic responses in approximately 30% of patients.[50,51] Omacetaxine mepesuccinate, a cephalotaxine ester and a derivative of homoharring-tonine that has excellent bioavailability through the subcutaneous route, is a multitar-geted protein synthase inhibitor that has been in clinical development for several years. Omacetaxine shows clinical activity against CML with a mechanism of action independent of tyrosine kinase inhibition and is not affected by the presence of mutations.[52,53] In a recently reported Phase 2 to 3 clinical study of omacetaxine administered at a dose of 1.25 mg/m^2 subcutaneously BID for 7 days (every 28 days) to 89 patients with CML (44 CP, 25 AP, and 20 BP) who are either intolerant or resistant to at least two TKIs (imatinib, dasatinib, or nilotinib), the rates of CHR and MCyR were 82% and 23% in CP, respectively.[54] In a similar trial enrolling 81 patients (49 CP, 17 AP, and 15 BP) with T315I mutation who did not respond to imatinib, omacetaxine led to a CHR in 86% and MCyR in 27% among patients treated in CCyR. These responses were durable.[55] The most commonly reported events were thrombocytopenia (58%); anemia (36%); and neutropenia (33%). Nonhematologic toxicities were primarily grade 1 to 2 with the most frequently reported events of diarrhea (44%); fatigue (35%); pyrexia (32%); nausea (26%); and asthenia (21%).

MUTATION STATUS AND CHOICE OF THERAPY

Although more than 100 BCR-ABL mutations have been identified in clinical samples,[18] the presence of a mutation does not typically lead to resistance. Baseline mutation screening for newly diagnosed patients with CML has shown no benefit for predicting response,[56] and should not be routinely used. In a study using highly sensitive DNA sequencing techniques, patients treated with imatinib showed no correlation between baseline mutation status and response, PFS, or OS. Other studies have confirmed that the identification of mutations pretherapy does not predict insensitivity to imatinib.[57–59]

The use of vitro mutation data to select a second-generation TKI remains a matter of controversy. In their seminal paper, Redaelli and colleagues[44] report on the in vitro activity of nilotinib, dasatinib, and bosutinib against 18 BCR-ABL mutations (**Table 3**). The eight most common mutations (T315I, Y253F/H, E255D/K/R/V, M351T, G250A/E, F359C/L/V, H396P/R, and M244V) found in 85% of patients with mutations were included in the analysis. The mutations were stratified using half maximal inhibitory concentration (IC$_{50}$) values into sensitive, moderately resistant, resistant, or highly resistant. The authors conclude that these data offer physicians a tool for selecting a patient-tailored TKI therapy. One of the major criticisms for using in vitro data in selecting the next line of therapy is that it does not fully predict the in vivo response.[60] In a recent publication, Laneuville and colleagues[60] report that adequate drug exposure to inhibit the BCR-ABL kinase located in the cytoplasm of leukemic cells requires satisfactory pharmacokinetics, which are affected by independent variables that might be related to molecular structure of the drug itself. They also note that the table as constructed in the article by Redaelli and colleagues[44] does not allow a side-by-side comparison of data, because columns for each inhibitor are normalized to the data within that column. Indeed, none of these studies take into account such factors as protein binding and cell influx and efflux or a variety of other in vivo factors that could affect results. Until more definitive results are published, treating physicians must not solely rely on in vitro data to select the next TKI for their patients who are imatinib-resistant or -intolerant.

Prospective clinical studies evaluating the choice of second-generation TKIs based on in vitro sensitivity data in imatinib-intolerant or -resistant patients are limited. In a retrospective analysis of 169 imatinib-resistant patients treated with a second-generation TKI at MDACC, 86 were found to have a mutation.[61] Forty-one patients were treated with dasatinib and 45 with nilotinib. Mutations were stratified on the basis of IC$_{50}$ values into high (n = 42); intermediate (n = 25); low (T315I, n = 9); and unknown (n = 10). Although response rates tended to be higher in patients

Table 3
In vitro sensitivity of different BCR-ABL mutants to different tyrosine kinase inhibitors

	IC$_{50}$-fold Increase (WT = 1)			
	Imatinib	Bosutinib	Dasatinib	Nilotinib
WT	1	1	1	1
L248V	3.54	2.97	5.11	2.80
G250E	6.86	4.31	4.45	4.56
Q252H	1.39	0.31	3.05	2.64
Y253F	3.58	0.96	1.58	3.23
E255K	6.02	9.47	5.61	6.69
E255V	16.99	5.53	3.44	10.31
D276G	2.18	0.60	1.44	2.00
E279K	3.55	0.95	1.64	2.05
V299L	1.54	26.10	8.65	1.34
T315I	17.50	45.42	75.03	39.41
F317L	2.60	2.42	4.46	2.22
M351T	1.76	0.70	0.88	0.44
F359V	2.86	0.93	1.49	5.16
L384M	1.28	0.47	2.21	2.33
H396P	2.43	0.43	1.07	2.41
H396R	3.91	0.81	1.63	3.10
G398R	0.35	1.16	0.69	0.49
F486S	8.10	2.31	3.04	1.85

Mutations can be classified as sensitive (IC$_{50}$ fold increase $\leq$2); resistant (between 2.01 and 10); or highly resistant (>10; T315I mutation).

without baseline mutations, there were no significant differences in CHR, MCyR, or CCyR between patients with and without baseline mutations. Response rates were higher in patients with CML-CP with low IC$_{50}$ mutations, compared with intermediate IC$_{50}$ mutations. The existence of a mutation at baseline was not shown to impact OS, but the presence of intermediate IC$_{50}$ mutations was significantly associated with poorer EFS (P = .0006) and OS (P = .03).

Among 1043 patients treated with second-line dasatinib in Phase 2 to 3 trials, 39% had a preexisting BCR-ABL mutation, including 48% of 805 patients with imatinib resistance or suboptimal response.[62] Sixty-three different BCR-ABL mutations affecting 49 amino acids were detected at baseline, with G250, M351, M244, and F359 most frequently affected. After 2 years of follow-up, dasatinib treatment of imatinib-resistant patients with or without a mutation resulted in notable response rates (CCyR, 43% vs 47%) and durable PFS (70% vs 80%). Impaired responses were observed with some mutations with a dasatinib median IC$_{50}$ greater than 3 nM; among patients with mutations with lower or unknown IC$_{50}$, efficacy was comparable with those with no mutation. In a subanalysis of a Phase II study of nilotinib in patients with imatinib-resistant or imatinib-intolerant CML-CP, baseline mutation data were assessed in 281 (88%) of 321 patients.[63] Among imatinib-resistant patients, the frequency of mutations at baseline was 55%. After 12 months of therapy, MCyR was achieved in 60%, CCyR in 40%, and MMR in 29% of patients without baseline mutations versus 49% (P = .145), 32% (P = .285), and 22% (P = .366), respectively, of patients with mutations. Patients with mutations that were less sensitive to nilotinib in vitro (IC_{50} >150 nM; Y253H, E255V/K, F359V/C) had less favorable responses; 13%, 43%, and 9% of patients with each of these mutations, respectively, achieved MCyR, and none achieved CCyR.

CURRENT RECOMMENDATIONS FOR TREATMENT OF CML

A proposed approach to the management of patients with CML is depicted in **Fig. 1**. Imatinib at a dose of 400 mg/day is considered the standard treatment. If patients do not achieve the landmarks as established by the ELN, modification to this therapy should be strongly considered. Dose escalation of imatinib can be considered, but is not likely to be effective in patients who never achieved a cytogenetic response on imatinib or those with known imatinib-resistant mutations. A change to a second-generation therapy may be a better option for most patients. In vitro and in vivo data have demonstrated that both dasatinib and nilotinib have a small and distinct set of mutants that confer decreased sensitivity: Y253H, E255K/V, and F359C/V for nilotinib and Q252H, E255K/V, V299L, and F317L for dasatinib. If the mutation analysis reveals any of these mutations, that particular second-generation TKI should be avoided.

For most patients who do not harbor a mutation, choice for a second-generation TKI is based on the presence of comorbid conditions. Dasatinib use is associated with the development of pleural and pericardial effusion,[64] bleeding,[65] and infection.[66] Caution should be exercised before prescribing dasatinib in patients with hypertension, asthma, pneumonia, gastrointestinal bleeding, chronic obstructive pulmonary disease, chest wall injury, congestive heart failure, autoimmune disorders, and concomitant aspirin use. Severe, uncontrolled diabetes and past pancreatitis are considered risk factors for nilotinib use because of the occurrence of grade 3 and 4

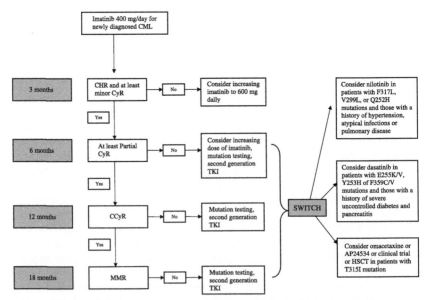

Fig. 1. A proposed schema for the management of patients with imatinib-resistant or imatinib-intolerant chronic-phase CML. CCyR, complete cytogenetic response; CHR, complete hematologic response; CyR, cytogenetic response; MMR, major molecular response; TKI, tyrosine kinase inhibitor.

lipase elevation (18%), bilirubin elevation (7%), and hyperglycemia (12%). QT prolongation is a concern with both agents, and the simultaneous use of agents prolonging the QT interval should be avoided. Although both dasatinib and nilotinib are ineffective against T315I *BCR-ABL*, this mutation is more likely to affect patients in the advanced phases of CML. Patients with T315I may achieve favorable outcomes with other therapies (eg, AP24534, omacetaxine). Stem cell transplant is generally reserved for patients who have not responded to a second- or third-generation TKI and for those patients with T315I mutation who have not responded to newer agents.

SUMMARY

Imatinib has dramatically altered the landscape of treatment for patients with CML. For most patients, the long-term outcomes including the PFS and OS are excellent. For a few subsets of patients who are intolerant or resistant to imatinib, newer second-generation TKIs are becoming excellent choices of therapy. The mechanisms of resistance, in vivo and in vitro sensitivities, and choice of agents are rapidly evolving. It is hoped that in the near future preclinical and clinical data will become available that will guide the treating physician to select the best TKI, both in the frontline and relapsed setting, for an individual patient with CML.

REFERENCES

1. Jemal A, Siegel R, Ward E, et al. Cancer statistics, 2009. CA Cancer J Clin 2009; 59:225–49.
2. Bartram CR, de Klein A, Hagemeijer A, et al. Translocation of c-ab1 oncogene correlates with the presence of a Philadelphia chromosome in chronic myelocytic leukaemia. Nature 1983;306:277–80.
3. Rowley JD. Letter: a new consistent chromosomal abnormality in chronic myelogenous leukaemia identified by quinacrine fluorescence and Giemsa staining. Nature 1973;243:290–3.
4. Druker BJ, Tamura S, Buchdunger E, et al. Effects of a selective inhibitor of the Abl tyrosine kinase on the growth of Bcr-Abl positive cells. Nat Med 1996;2:561–6.
5. Druker BJ, Talpaz M, Resta DJ, et al. Efficacy and safety of a specific inhibitor of the BCR-ABL tyrosine kinase in chronic myeloid leukemia. N Engl J Med 2001; 344:1031–7.
6. Kantarjian H, Sawyers C, Hochhaus A, et al. Hematologic and cytogenetic responses to imatinib mesylate in chronic myelogenous leukemia. N Engl J Med 2002;346:645–52.
7. O'Brien SG, Guilhot F, Larson RA, et al. Imatinib compared with interferon and low-dose cytarabine for newly diagnosed chronic-phase chronic myeloid leukemia. N Engl J Med 2003;348:994–1004.
8. Deininger M, O'Brien SG, Guilhot F, et al. International randomized study of Interferon Vs STI571 (IRIS) 8-year follow up: sustained survival and low risk for progression or events in patients with newly diagnosed chronic myeloid leukemia in chronic phase (CML-CP) treated with imatinib. (ASH Annual Meeting Abstracts). Blood 2009;114:1126.
9. Zhang WW, Cortes JE, Yao H, et al. Predictors of primary imatinib resistance in chronic myelogenous leukemia are distinct from those in secondary imatinib resistance. J Clin Oncol 2009;27:3642–9.
10. le Coutre P, Tassi E, Varella-Garcia M, et al. Induction of resistance to the Abelson inhibitor STI571 in human leukemic cells through gene amplification. Blood 2000; 95:1758–66.

11. Gorre ME, Mohammed M, Ellwood K, et al. Clinical resistance to STI-571 cancer therapy caused by BCR-ABL gene mutation or amplification. Science 2001;293: 876–80.

12. Weisberg E, Griffin JD. Mechanism of resistance to the ABL tyrosine kinase inhibitor STI571 in BCR/ABL-transformed hematopoietic cell lines. Blood 2000;95: 3498–505.

13. Branford S, Rudzki Z, Walsh S, et al. Detection of BCR-ABL mutations in patients with CML treated with imatinib is virtually always accompanied by clinical resistance, and mutations in the ATP phosphate-binding loop (P-loop) are associated with a poor prognosis. Blood 2003;102:276–83.

14. Hochhaus A, Kreil S, Corbin AS, et al. Molecular and chromosomal mechanisms of resistance to imatinib (STI571) therapy. Leukemia 2002;16:2190–6.

15. Corbin AS, La Rosee P, Stoffregen EP, et al. Several Bcr-Abl kinase domain mutants associated with imatinib mesylate resistance remain sensitive to imatinib. Blood 2003;101:4611–4.

16. Soverini S, Colarossi S, Gnani A, et al. Contribution of ABL kinase domain mutations to imatinib resistance in different subsets of Philadelphia-positive patients: by the GIMEMA Working Party on Chronic Myeloid Leukemia. Clin Cancer Res 2006;12:7374–9.

17. Jabbour E, Kantarjian H, Jones D, et al. Long-term incidence and outcome of BCR-ABL mutations in patients (pts) with chronic myeloid leukemia (CML) treated with imatinib mesylate P-loop mutations are not associated with worse outcome. (ASH Annual Meeting Abstracts). Blood 2004;104:1007.

18. Jabbour E, Kantarjian H, Jones D, et al. Frequency and clinical significance of BCR-ABL mutations in patients with chronic myeloid leukemia treated with imatinib mesylate. Leukemia 2006;20:1767–73.

19. Soverini S, Martinelli G, Amabile M, et al. Denaturing-HPLC-based assay for detection of ABL mutations in chronic myeloid leukemia patients resistant to imatinib. Clin Chem 2004;50:1205–13.

20. Deininger MW, McGreevey L, Willis S, et al. Detection of ABL kinase domain mutations with denaturing high-performance liquid chromatography. Leukemia 2004;18:864–71.

21. Apperley JF. Part I: mechanisms of resistance to imatinib in chronic myeloid leukaemia. Lancet Oncol 2007;8:1018–29.

22. Hochhaus A, La Rosee P. Imatinib therapy in chronic myelogenous leukemia: strategies to avoid and overcome resistance. Leukemia 2004;18:1321–31.

23. Version 2. National Comprehensive Cancer Network. Clinical Practice Guidelines in Oncology; 2010.

24. Baccarani M, Cortes J, Pane F, et al. Chronic myeloid leukemia: an update of concepts and management recommendations of European LeukemiaNet. J Clin Oncol 2009;27:6041–51.

25. Press RD, Willis SG, Laudadio J, et al. Determining the rise in BCR-ABL RNA that optimally predicts a kinase domain mutation in patients with chronic myeloid leukemia on imatinib. Blood 2009;114:2598–605.

26. Kantarjian HM, Larson RA, Guilhot F, et al. Efficacy of imatinib dose escalation in patients with chronic myeloid leukemia in chronic phase. Cancer 2009;115: 551–60.

27. Jabbour E, Kantarjian HM, Jones D, et al. Imatinib mesylate dose escalation is associated with durable responses in patients with chronic myeloid leukemia after cytogenetic failure on standard-dose imatinib therapy. Blood 2009;113: 2154–60.

28. Cortes JE, Kantarjian HM, Goldberg SL, et al. High-dose imatinib in newly diagnosed chronic-phase chronic myeloid leukemia: high rates of rapid cytogenetic and molecular responses. J Clin Oncol 2009;27:4754–9.

29. Baccarani M, Druker BJ, Cortes-Franco J, et al. 24 months update of the TOPS study: a phase III, of 400mg/d (SD-IM) versus 800mg/d (HD-IM) of imatinib mesylate (IM) in patients (Pts) with newly diagnosed, previously untreated chronic myeloid leukemia in chronic phase (CML-CP). (ASH Annual Meeting Abstracts). Blood 2009;114:337.

30. Baccarani M, Rosti G, Castagnetti F, et al. Comparison of imatinib 400 mg and 800 mg daily in the front-line treatment of high-risk, Philadelphia-positive chronic myeloid leukemia: a European LeukemiaNet Study. Blood 2009;113:4497–504.

31. Lombardo LJ, Lee FY, Chen P, et al. Discovery of N-(2-chloro-6-methyl- phenyl)-2-(6-(4-(2-hydroxyethyl)- piperazin-1-yl)-2-methylpyrimidin-4- ylamino)thiazole-5-carboxamide (BMS-354825), a dual Src/Abl kinase inhibitor with potent antitumor activity in preclinical assays. J Med Chem 2004;47:6658–61.

32. Cortes J, Rousselot P, Kim DW, et al. Dasatinib induces complete hematologic and cytogenetic responses in patients with imatinib-resistant or -intolerant chronic myeloid leukemia in blast crisis. Blood 2007;109:3207–13.

33. Guilhot F, Apperley J, Kim DW, et al. Dasatinib induces significant hematologic and cytogenetic responses in patients with imatinib-resistant or -intolerant chronic myeloid leukemia in accelerated phase. Blood 2007;109:4143–50.

34. Hochhaus A, Baccarani M, Deininger M, et al. Dasatinib induces durable cytogenetic responses in patients with chronic myelogenous leukemia in chronic phase with resistance or intolerance to imatinib. Leukemia 2008;22:1200–6.

35. Shah NP, Kantarjian HM, Kim DW, et al. Intermittent target inhibition with dasatinib 100 mg once daily preserves efficacy and improves tolerability in imatinib-resistant and -intolerant chronic-phase chronic myeloid leukemia. J Clin Oncol 2008;26:3204–12.

36. Cortes JE, Jones D, O'Brien S, et al. Results of dasatinib therapy in patients with early chronic-phase chronic myeloid leukemia. J Clin Oncol 2010;28:398–404.

37. Golemovic M, Verstovsek S, Giles F, et al. AMN107, a novel aminopyrimidine inhibitor of Bcr-Abl, has in vitro activity against imatinib-resistant chronic myeloid leukemia. Clin Cancer Res 2005;11:4941–7.

38. Weisberg E, Manley PW, Breitenstein W, et al. Characterization of AMN107, a selective inhibitor of native and mutant Bcr-Abl. Cancer Cell 2005;7:129–41.

39. Hocchaus A, Cortes J, Appereley J, et al. Nilotinib in chronic myeloid leukemia patients in accelerated phase (CML-AP) with imatinib resistance or intolerance: 24-month follow-up results of a phase 2 study [abstract 0631]. Haematologica 2009;94(Suppl 2).

40. Kantarjian HM, Giles FJ, Bhalla KN, et al. Update on imatinib-resistant chronic myeloid leukemia patients in chronic phase (CML-CP) on nilotinib therapy at 24 months: clinical response, safety, and long-term outcomes. ASH Annual Meeting Abstracts 2009;114:1129.

41. Cortes JE, Jones D, O'Brien S, et al. Nilotinib as front-line treatment for patients with chronic myeloid leukemia in early chronic phase. J Clin Oncol 2010;28:392–7.

42. O'Dwyer MC, Kent E, Parker M, et al. Nilotinib 300 mg twice daily is effective and well tolerated as first line treatment of Ph-positive chronic myeloid leukemia in chronic phase: preliminary results of the ICORG 0802 phase 2 study. ASH Annual Meeting Abstracts 2009;114:3294.

43. Rosti G, Palandri F, Castagnetti F, et al. Nilotinib for the frontline treatment of Ph(+) chronic myeloid leukemia. Blood 2009;114:4933–8.

44. Redaelli S, Piazza R, Rostagno R, et al. Activity of bosutinib, dasatinib, and nilotinib against 18 imatinib-resistant BCR/ABL mutants. J Clin Oncol 2009;27:469–71.
45. Cortes J, Kantarjian HM, Kim DW, et al. Efficacy and safety of bosutinib (SKI-606) in patients with chronic phase (CP) Ph+ chronic myelogenous leukemia (CML) with resistance or intolerance to imatinib. (ASH Annual Meeting Abstracts). Blood 2008;112:1098.
46. Gambacorti-Passerini C, Kantarjian H, Bruemmendorf T, et al. Bosutinib (SKI-606) demonstrates clinical activity and is well tolerated among patients with AP and BP CML and Ph+ ALL. (ASH Annual Meeting Abstracts). Blood 2007;110:473.
47. O'Hare T, Shakespeare WC, Zhu X, et al. AP24534, a pan-BCR-ABL inhibitor for chronic myeloid leukemia, potently inhibits the T315I mutant and overcomes mutation-based resistance. Cancer Cell 2009;16:401–12.
48. Cortes J, Talpaz M, Deininger M, et al. A Phase 1 trial of oral AP24534 in patients with refractory chronic myeloid leukemia and other hematologic malignancies: first results of safety and clinical activity against T315I and resistant mutations. (ASH Annual Meeting Abstracts). Blood 2009;114:643.
49. Cortes J, Paquette R, Talpaz M, et al. Preliminary clinical activity in a Phase I trial of the BCR-ABL/IGF- 1R/aurora kinase inhibitor XL228 in patients with Ph++ leukemias with either failure to multiple TKI therapies or with T315I mutation. (ASH Annual Meeting Abstracts). Blood 2008;112:3232.
50. O'Brien S, Kantarjian H, Koller C, et al. Sequential homoharringtonine and interferon-alpha in the treatment of early chronic phase chronic myelogenous leukemia. Blood 1999;93:4149–53.
51. O'Brien S, Talpaz M, Cortes J, et al. Simultaneous homoharringtonine and interferon-alpha in the treatment of patients with chronic-phase chronic myelogenous leukemia. Cancer 2002;94:2024–32.
52. Kantarjian HM, Talpaz M, Santini V, et al. Homoharringtonine: history, current research, and future direction. Cancer 2001;92:1591–605.
53. O'Brien S, Kantarjian H, Keating M, et al. Homoharringtonine therapy induces responses in patients with chronic myelogenous leukemia in late chronic phase. Blood 1995;86:3322–6.
54. Cortes-Franco J, Raghunadharao D, Parikh P, et al. Safety and efficacy of subcutaneous-administered omacetaxine mepesuccinate in chronic myeloid leukemia (CML) patients who are resistant or intolerant to two or more tyrosine kinase inhibitors: results of a multicenter Phase 2/3 study. (ASH Annual Meeting Abstracts). Blood 2009;114:861.
55. Cortes-Franco J, Khoury HJ, Nicolini FE, et al. Safety and efficacy of subcutaneous-administered omacetaxine mepesuccinate in imatinib-resistant chronic myeloid leukemia (CML) patients who harbor the Bcr- Abl T315I mutation-results of an ongoing multicenter Phase 2/3 study. (ASH Annual Meeting Abstracts). Blood 2009;114:644.
56. Willis SG, Lange T, Demehri S, et al. High-sensitivity detection of BCR-ABL kinase domain mutations in imatinib-naive patients: correlation with clonal cytogenetic evolution but not response to therapy. Blood 2005;106:2128–37.
57. Khorashad JS, Anand M, Marin D, et al. The presence of a BCR-ABL mutant allele in CML does not always explain clinical resistance to imatinib. Leukemia 2006;20:658–63.
58. Mauro MJ. Mutational analysis and overcoming imatinib resistance in chronic myeloid leukemia with novel tyrosine kinase inhibitors. Curr Treat Options Oncol 2007;8:287–95.

59. Sherbenou DW, Wong MJ, Humayun A, et al. Mutations of the BCR-ABL-kinase domain occur in a minority of patients with stable complete cytogenetic response to imatinib. Leukemia 2007;21:489–93.
60. Laneuville P, Dilea C, Yin OQ, et al. Comparative In vitro cellular data alone are insufficient to predict clinical responses and guide the choice of BCR-ABL inhibitor for treating imatinib-resistant chronic myeloid leukemia. J Clin Oncol 2010;28: e169–71 [author reply: e172].
61. Jabbour E, Jones D, Kantarjian HM, et al. Long-term outcome of patients with chronic myeloid leukemia treated with second-generation tyrosine kinase inhibitors after imatinib failure is predicted by the in vitro sensitivity of BCR-ABL kinase domain mutations. Blood 2009;114:2037–43.
62. Muller MC, Cortes JE, Kim DW, et al. Dasatinib treatment of chronic-phase chronic myeloid leukemia: analysis of responses according to preexisting BCR-ABL mutations. Blood 2009;114:4944–53.
63. Hughes T, Saglio G, Branford S, et al. Impact of baseline BCR-ABL mutations on response to nilotinib in patients with chronic myeloid leukemia in chronic phase. J Clin Oncol 2009;27:4204–10.
64. Quintas-Cardama A, Kantarjian H, O'Brien S, et al. Pleural effusion in patients with chronic myelogenous leukemia treated with dasatinib after imatinib failure. J Clin Oncol 2007;25:3908–14.
65. Quintas-Cardama A, Kantarjian H, Ravandi F, et al. Bleeding diathesis in patients with chronic myelogenous leukemia receiving dasatinib therapy. Cancer 2009; 115:2482–90.
66. Sillaber C, Herrmann H, Bennett K, et al. Immunosuppression and atypical infections in CML patients treated with dasatinib at 140 mg daily. Eur J Clin Invest 2009;39:1098–109.

BCR-ABL Mutations in Chronic Myeloid Leukemia

Thomas Ernst, Dr. med[a], Paul La Rosée, Dr. med[a],
Martin C. Müller, Dr. med[b], Andreas Hochhaus, Dr. med[a],*

KEYWORDS

- Chronic myeloid leukemia • Imatinib • BCR-ABL mutations

Crystallographic analysis has shown that imatinib binds to and stabilizes an inactive conformation of ABL, in which the centrally located activation loop is not phosphorylated and thus in a closed position.[1] Before first clinical reports of resistance due to kinase mutations, biochemical studies guided by the crystallographic analysis predicted mutant BCR-ABL with retained kinase activity, but reduced or lost drug affinity to imatinib as a potential mechanism of resistance.[2] Consistent with preclinical analysis, Gorre and colleagues[3] found that imatinib resistance was associated with the reactivation of BCR-ABL signal transduction in a cohort of relapsed patients. The exchange of the amino acids threonine and isoleucine at position 315 (T315I) of the BCR-ABL protein was the first mutation detected in imatinib resistant chronic myeloid leukemia (CML) patients. Sequencing of cloning products revealed the T315I mutation in 6 of 9 resistant patients. Based on the known crystal structure of the ABL kinase domain, this substitution was predicted to abrogate affinity for the drug. Since this original report, many investigators have reported kinase domain mutations that impart resistance to imatinib.[4–6]

A bacterial mutagenesis screen revealed a set of mutations that grow out in the presence of imatinib.[7] These mutations largely reflected the findings in clinical trials. Mutations may be categorized into 4 groups, based upon the crystallographic structure of ABL: (1) those that directly impair imatinib binding to the catalytic domain of the oncogenic protein; (2) those within the P-loop; (3) those within the activation loop, preventing the kinase from achieving the inactive conformation required for imatinib binding; and (4) those within the catalytic domain with impact on the activity of the tyrosine kinase. Even mutations outside the kinase domain can lead to enhanced autophosphorylation of the kinase, thereby stabilizing the active conformation that resists imatinib binding. Mutant BCR-ABL alleles retain biologic activity but show varying degrees of resistance

[a] Klinik für Innere Medizin II, Universitätsklinikum Jena, Erlanger Allee 101, 07740 Jena, Germany
[b] III. Medizinische Klinik, Universitätsmedizin Mannheim, Theodor-Kutzer-Ufer 1-3, 68167 Mannheim, Germany
* Corresponding author. Erlanger Allee 101, 07740 Jena, Germany.
E-mail address: andreas.hochhaus@med.uni-jena.de

Hematol Oncol Clin N Am 25 (2011) 997–1008
doi:10.1016/j.hoc.2011.09.005
0889-8588/11/$ – see front matter © 2011 Elsevier Inc. All rights reserved.

to imatinib in biochemical and cellular assays.[8] However, the level of resistance against imatinib in vitro cannot always explain resistance seen in patients.

METHODS OF BCR-ABL MUTATION DETECTION

Several techniques have been described for the detection of BCR-ABL kinase domain mutations, but there is currently no consensus concerning which technique should be used (**Table 1**). Mutations can be reliably and sensitively detected by selection and expansion of specific clones followed by DNA sequencing.[3,9] This procedure, however, is cumbersome and not eligible for clinical routine. Alternatively, sequencing of nested polymerase chain reaction (PCR)-amplified BCR-ABL products has been widely used to search for known and unknown BCR-ABL kinase domain mutations.[6,10] A potential limitation of direct sequencing is the sensitivity of only 10% to 20%. Sensitivities of 1% to 5% could be obtained by double-gradient denaturing electrophoresis,[11] pyrosequencing,[12] high-resolution melting,[13] or array based assays.[14,15] More sensitive methods include peptide nucleic acid-based PCR clamping[16] and allele-specific oligonucleotide (ASO-) PCR.[17–21] However, these techniques are specific and cannot be applied for screening of unknown mutations. Denaturing high-performance liquid chromatography (D-HPLC) has been described as a highly sensitive screening method for BCR-ABL kinase domain mutations, even when the site of the mutation is unknown.[22–25]

Use of various techniques for the detection of BCR-ABL mutations has led to different frequencies of mutations that are reported. Furthermore, the pattern of individual mutations reported seems to depend on the specific method used for mutation detection. Standardized techniques and protocols for the detection of BCR-ABL mutations will be necessary to obtain comparable mutation results within clinical studies. A recent cooperative evaluation of different methods of detecting BCR-ABL kinase domain mutations in 3 European laboratories has revealed major differences particularly in the detection of low-level mutations (ie, mutations below the sensitivity of standard direct sequencing).[26] Further studies toward standardized techniques and protocols are necessary and underway.

BCR-ABL MUTATION TYPES
BCR-ABL Point Mutations

More than 70 amino acid residues within the kinase domain have been reported as targets of about 100 different mutations. Recently published review articles have

Table 1		
Methods for the detection of BCR-ABL kinase domain mutations		
Sensitivity	**Method**	**References**
10%–20%	Selection of clones plus DNA sequencing	3,9
	Nested polymerase chain reaction (PCR) plus DNA sequencing	6,10
1%–5%	Denaturing high-performance liquid chromatography (D-HPLC)	22–25
	Double gradient denaturing electrophoresis	11
	Pyrosequencing	12
	High-resolution melting (HRM)	13
	MALDI-TOF mass spectrometry	14
	Nanofluidic array	15
<1%	Fluorescence PCR and PNA clamping	16
	Allele-specific oligonucleotide (ASO-) PCR	17–21

summarized the distribution and relative sensitivities to imatinib in vitro.[27,28] Most reported mutants are rare, whereas 7 mutated sites comprise two-thirds of all mutations detected: G250, Y253, E255, T315, M351, F359, H396. Different amino acid substitutions occur at the same residue (eg, F317C, F317L, and F317V) and confer different imatinib sensitivities. The functional importance of individual amino acid substitutions with regard to oncogenicity of BCR-ABL is difficult to determine. Besides being gain of function or loss of function mutations, they might simply be regarded as surrogate markers of the increased genetic instability associated with advanced phase disease. Griswold and colleagues[29] studied the transformation potential, kinase activity, and substrate specificity of five of the most frequent mutations—Y253F, E255K, T315I, M351T, and H396P. Compared with unmutated BCR-ABL, Y253F was noted to produce enhanced kinase activity (gain of function), with E255K producing comparable activity. The remaining 3 mutations decreased enzymatic function (loss of function). Transforming potency did not always correlate with kinase activity. However, clear differences did exist in the pan-tyrosine phosphorylation patterns of the Ba/F3 cells expressing the various mutants, which would be consistent with differences in substrate use and signaling pathway activation. Phosphoproteomic studies on mutant T315I also support the notion of mutation-dependent oncogenic potential of individual substitutions.[30] Skaggs and colleagues showed that the intramolecular tyrosine phosphorylation pattern is altered, indicating modified biologic activity of mutant BCR-ABL.

BCR-ABL Deletion Mutants

Some imatinib resistant patients express deletion mutants of BCR-ABL, apparently due to mis-splicing. Most commonly these deletion mutants lack a significant proportion of the kinase domain that includes the P-loop.[31] The L248V mutation was shown in 2 patients to additionally induce the alternative splicing of a shorter variant by introducing a donor splice site within ABL exon 4 lacking amino acids 248 to 274. Sherbenou and colleagues[32] performed a screen for such mutations in 95 patients with CML and identified 14 patients (15%) with a total of six different deletion mutations. Deletion mutants detected most frequently involved splice junctions. Functional studies further demonstrated that such deletion mutations are not oncogenic and are catalytically inactive. The authors hypothesized that coexpressing BCR-ABL deletion mutants have a dominant-negative effect on the native form through heterocomplex formation. However, the prognostic impact of coexpression of deletion mutants in CML patients during imatinib treatment is unknown.

ABL Polymorphisms

The BCR-ABL[K247R] change is based on a rare single-nucleotide polymorphism (SNP) of ABL occurring likewise in healthy controls and nonhematologic cell types.[33] Despite its juxtaposition to the P-loop, functional analysis showed no alteration compared with nonmutated BCR-ABL. To investigate if other changes in the BCR-ABL kinase domain should be considered as SNPs rather than acquired mutations, 911 CML patients after failure or suboptimal response to imatinib were screened for BCR-ABL kinase domain mutations.[34] SNP analysis was based on the search for nucleotide changes in corresponding normal, nontranslocated ABL alleles by ABL allele-specific PCR following mutation analysis. In addition to the K247R polymorphism five new SNPs within the BCR-ABL kinase domain were uncovered; two of them led to amino acid changes (**Table 2**). SNPs theoretically could modify the primary response to tyrosine kinase inhibitors, and must therefore be distinguished from acquired mutations that govern the evolution of secondary resistance. Novel point mutations should be confirmed by analyzing the normal ABL alleles to exclude polymorphisms.

Table 2
Polymorphisms within the BCR-ABL kinase domain in 911 analyzed chronic myeloid leukemia patients

Nucleotide Position[a]	Nucleotide Polymorphism	Amino Acid Change[b]	N[c]	Allele Frequency (%)
58,758	A	T240T	1	0.1
58,778	G	K247R	9	1.0
68,708	G	F311V	2	0.2
68,722	G	T315T	1	0.1
68,736	G	Y320C	1	0.1
74,901	G	E499E	73	8.0

[a] Nucleotide positions according to GenBank accession number U07563 for the ABL 1a splice variant.
[b] Amino acid residues are denoted with the single letter code and correspond to the ABL 1a variant.
[c] Total number of patients harboring the respective polymorphism.

Data from Ernst T, Hoffmann J, Erben P, et al. ABL single nucleotide polymorphisms may masquerade as BCR-ABL mutations associated with resistance to tyrosine kinase inhibitors in patients with chronic myeloid leukemia. Haematologica 2008;93:1389–93.

INCIDENCE OF BCR-ABL MUTATIONS

The frequency of BCR-ABL mutations in resistant patients was reported to range from 42% to 90% depending on the methodology of detection, the definition of resistance, and the phase of the disease.[9,35] Mutations are found more frequently in accelerated phase or blast crisis. A twofold increase of the BCR-ABL transcript level might be a diagnostic red flag to detect patients carrying resistance mutations.[36] The identification of the specific type of mutation in relapsed patients is of prognostic relevance, since the different types of mutation correlate with the risk of evolution of relapsed patients.[37] However, mutant Ph+ subclones may remain at low levels, may be transient or unstable, or may not be consistently associated with subsequent relapse.[12] In many cases, mutations have been detected in samples that were collected during imatinib treatment, but in several cases mutations were also traced back to samples collected prior to treatment, especially in patients who consecutively developed accelerated phase or blast crisis.[19,38] Using more sensitive techniques, mutations were also found in imatinib-naïve patients and in patients having achieved complete cytogenetic remission.[39] It is important to note that Ph+ primitive cells have been reported to be less sensitive to imatinib in vitro and in vivo, to harbor BCR-ABL mutations even prior to imatinib exposure, and to rapidly develop mutations under imatinib-induced selection pressure.[40,41] Various BCR-ABL mutations show different biochemical and clinical properties. The biochemical and cellular impact of different mutations is heterogeneous, ranging from a minor increase of the median inhibitory concentrations of imatinib to a virtual insensitivity of imatinib.[8] The T315I mutation and some mutations affecting the so-called P-loop of BCR-ABL confer a greater level of resistance, whereas the biochemical resistance of other mutations can be overcome by dose increase, and others seem functionally irrelevant.[37,42] Thus, the detection of a kinase domain mutation must be interpreted within the clinical context.

DYNAMICS OF BCR-ABL MUTATIONS DURING IMATINIB TREATMENT

Results from in vitro models predicted most of the resistance mutations that were detected later on in clinical trials with different kinase inhibitors.[7,43,44] The sensitivity of mutant BCR-ABL to tyrosine kinase inhibitors can be estimated by the respective inhibitory concentration for 50% in vitro inhibition (IC_{50}), determined either in cellular or biochemical assays. It has been suggested to modify the clinical strategy in resistant patients with a kinase domain mutation on the basis of the IC_{50} determined in vitro.[28,45] Mutations with low-level resistance according to this model might be amenable to dose increase. Mutations with intermediate resistance on the other hand might call for second-line treatment with dasatinib or nilotinib, depending on the individual sensitivity to the tyrosine kinase inhibitor (**Table 3**). In the case of the pan-resistant T315I mutation shown to be associated with a poor prognosis in an international registry database, allogeneic stem cell transplantation or experimental treatment needs to be considered.[46–48] It is, however, important to note that a mutation detected in patients should be linked to functional in vitro data, as mutations may truly be the cause of resistance. Others may represent innocent bystanders that accompany other mechanisms of resistance. A comprehensive list of the in vitro IC_{50} - values to various tyrosine kinase inhibitors was published recently.[45] Clearly, the in vitro prediction of tyrosine kinase inhibitor activity not necessarily reflect the complexity of tyrosine kinase inhibitor activity in vivo, which is also dependent on pharmacokinetics, tissue distribution and washout, cellular availability, or other difficult-to-determine factors.[49]

The authors investigated the dynamics of mutated clones in CML patients prior to relapse in 95 patients by D-HPLC and direct sequencing.[25] In patients harboring mutations, hematologic relapse occurred after a median of 12.9 months (range, 0.9–44.2 months). The median time to first detection of BCR-ABL mutations was 5.8 months (range, 0–30.5 months) after starting imatinib therapy. The median interval of mutation detection and hematologic relapse correlated with the degree of resistance of the mutated clone to imatinib, expressed as the increase of the IC_{50}. Nine patients showed evidence of BCR-ABL mutations prior to imatinib therapy (T315I, n = 4; M351T, n = 3; M244V and Y253H, n = 1 each). The sensitive detection of small numbers of mutated clones could provide clinical benefit by triggering early therapeutic interventions.

Another study published by Khorashad and colleagues[50] reported systematic and regular analysis of mutations by conventional sequencing in a cohort of 319 chronic-phase CML patients who were treated with imatinib. The authors reported

Table 3
Resistance and intermediate sensitivity of mutations to nilotinib (IC_{50}>150 nM) and dasatinib (IC_{50}>3 nM)

	Nilotinib	Dasatinib
Resistance	T315I	T315I
Intermediate sensitivity	Y253H	L248V
	E255K/V	G250E
	F359C/V	Q252H
		E255K/V
		V299L
		F317L
		L384M
		F486S

Data from Müller MC, Cortes JE, Kim DW, et al. Dasatinib treatment of chronic-phase chronic myeloid leukemia: analysis of responses according to preexisting BCR-ABL mutations. Blood 2009;114:4944–53; Hughes T, Saglio G, Branford S, et al. Impact of baseline BCR-ABL mutations on response to nilotinib in patients with chronic myeloid leukemia in chronic phase. J Clin Oncol 2009;27:4204–10.

a 5-year cumulative incidence of mutations of 6.6% and 17% for early and late chronic phase, respectively. Of the 319 patients, 214 (67%) achieved complete cytogenetic remission. The identification of a mutation without other evidence of imatinib resistance was highly predictive for loss of complete cytogenetic remission and for progression to advanced phase, although the intervals from first identification to loss of complete cytogenetic remission and disease progression were relatively long (median 21 and 16 months, respectively). Mutations in the P-loop were associated with a higher risk of progression than mutations elsewhere.

Looking exclusively at patients with stable complete cytogenetic response, Sherbenou and colleagues[51] demonstrated mutations in 8 of 42 (19%) cases. Four patients with mutations had a concomitant rise of BCR-ABL transcript levels, two of whom subsequently relapsed; the remaining four did not have an increase in transcript levels, and follow-up samples, when amplifiable, showed native BCR-ABL. Thus, BCR-ABL-kinase domain mutations in patients with a stable complete cytogenetic remission are infrequent, and their detection does not consistently predict relapse.

The same group reported a study on 66 consecutive unselected CML patients.[19] They found correlations between the pretreatment presence of low-level mutations, and both stage of disease and clonal cytogenetic evolution, but not with the probability of response to imatinib. ASO-PCR detected BCR-ABL kinase domain mutations in a significant proportion of CML patients with advanced disease, but not in the chronic phase. Not all of the mutant clones were selected in the presence of imatinib. Even the completely resistant T315I mutant, when detected at a low level prior to treatment, did not prove to be selected on treatment. Consistent with this, Korashad and colleagues[12] showed a lack of correlation between the residual disease and the presence of a predominant kinase domain mutation in a cohort of early and late chronic phase CML patients. This suggests that other factors must be operational to modulate resistance in mutant carrying clones.[52] As a practical consequence, screening with high sensitivity methods for low-level kinase domain mutations in newly diagnosed patients is not recommended for clinical routine. The long term significance of pretreatment low-level mutations still needs to be assessed prospectively.

In contrast to chronic phase CML, BCR-ABL mutations are common in Ph+ acute lymphoblastic leukemia (ALL) patients at diagnosis prior to imatinib therapy. Using D-HPLC and ASO-PCR, BCR-ABL mutations were detected in 40% of newly diagnosed, imatinib-naïve Ph+ ALL patients.[53] At relapse, the dominant cell clone harbored an identical mutation in 90% of cases; the overall prevalence of mutations at relapse was 80%. P-loop mutations predominated and were not associated with an inferior hematologic or molecular remission rate or shorter remission duration compared with unmutated BCR-ABL. BCR-ABL mutations conferring high-level imatinib resistance were present in a substantial proportion of patients with de novo Ph+ ALL and eventually gave rise to relapse.

DYNAMICS OF BCR-ABL MUTATIONS AFTER IMATINIB CESSATION

Before the advent of second-generation tyrosine kinase inhibitors, patients with resistance to imatinib were treated with nonspecific drugs, like hydroxyurea. After stopping imatinib due to a lack of efficacy in the case of a BCR-ABL mutation, absolute and relative reduction of the mutated clone has been observed in the majority of patients.[54,55] This might be explained by the proliferative advantage of clones harboring unmutated BCR-ABL in the absence of the selective pressure of tyrosine kinase inhibitors. Deselection of mutant BCR-ABL positive clones after cessation of tyrosine kinase inhibitor therapy is a common and reproducible phenomenon.

However, BCR-ABL^{T315I} clones tend to account for a persisting proportion of BCR-ABL expression after cessation, although decreasing in size due to a gradually declining BCR-ABL ratio. The reduction of the proportion of BCR-ABL^{T315I} expression under the threshold of detection might offer the therapeutic option to resume at least temporarily a tyrosine kinase inhibitor treatment.[55] Quantification of the mutated clone to evaluate treatment efficacy should consider the total BCR-ABL load (ie, the proportion of mutated BCR-ABL in total BCR-ABL should be multiplied by the BCR-ABL transcript level).

Omacetaxine (Homoharringtonine, HHT), a cephalotaxine ester that has demonstrated clinical activity in CML, inhibits protein synthesis and induces cell differentiation and apoptosis. The absence of cross-resistance between HHT and imatinib in resistant leukemic cell lines has been demonstrated, and a possible synergy between the 2 compounds has been observed in vitro.[56] BCR-ABL^{T315I} may completely disappear during treatment with HHT, even after persistence of the clone during hydroxyurea therapy.[57]

DYNAMICS OF BCR-ABL MUTATIONS DURING DASATINIB AND NILOTINIB THERAPY

Dasatinib is a thiazolecarboxamide that is structurally unrelated to imatinib. Cocrystal analysis has shown that the compound binds to the ABL kinase domain in the active (open) conformation and also inhibits SRC family kinases. Preclinical studies have revealed the compound to be approximately 300-fold more potent than imatinib and to harbor potent inhibitory activity against nearly all imatinib-resistant mutants tested.[58] Nilotinib is an aminopyrimidine that is a structural derivative of imatinib. Like imatinib, nilotinib binds the ABL kinase domain in the inactive conformation, but with more ABL-specific and powerful potency relative to imatinib. Importantly, this compound harbors activity against most imatinib-resistant mutations tested.[59]

Ethyl-N-nitrosourea (ENU)-exposed Ba/F3-p210$^{BCR-ABL}$ cells were used to compare incidence and types of kinase domain mutants emerging in the presence of imatinib, dasatinib, and nilotinib, alone and in dual combinations.[44] Twenty different mutations were identified with imatinib, 10 with nilotinib and nine with dasatinib. At intermediate drug levels, the spectrum narrowed to F317V and T315I for dasatinib and Y253H, E255V, and T315I for nilotinib. Cross-resistance in vitro is limited to T315I, which is also the only mutant isolated at drug concentrations equivalent to maximally achievable plasma trough levels. With drug combinations, maximal suppression of resistant clone outgrowth was achieved at lower concentrations compared with single agents, suggesting that such combinations may be equipotent to higher-dose single agents. Through saturation mutagenesis, 10 BCR-ABL mutations resistant to dasatinib were identified, eight of which occurred at drug contact residues. The combination of imatinib plus dasatinib greatly reduced the recovery of drug-resistant clones.[60]

To identify mutations in BCR-ABL that could result in resistance to nilotinib, a cDNA library of BCR-ABL mutants was introduced into Ba/F3 cells followed by selection in nilotinib.[61] A total of 46 out of 86 colonies had single-point mutations in BCR-ABL, with a total of 17 different mutations, all within the kinase domain. Each of the 17 single-point mutants was reconstructed by site directed mutagenesis of native BCR-ABL and found to be approximately 2.5- to 800-fold more resistant to nilotinib than native BCR-ABL. The mutations included six known imatinib-resistant mutations, including T315I, which showed complete resistance to nilotinib. Most nilotinib-resistant mutants were also resistant to imatinib.

Analysis of BCR-ABL in patients who relapsed after sequential treatment with the ABL inhibitors imatinib and dasatinib revealed evolving resistant BCR-ABL kinase domain mutations in all cases.[62] Twelve patients relapsed with the pan-resistant T315I mutation, whereas 6 patients developed novel BCR-ABL mutations predicted to retain sensitivity to imatinib based on in vitro studies. Selection for compound mutants (ie, two or more BCR-ABL mutations in the same molecule) can substantially limit the potential effectiveness of retreating patients with inhibitors that have previously failed. These findings demonstrate the potential hazards of sequential kinase inhibitor therapy and suggest a role for a combination of ABL kinase inhibitors to prevent the outgrowth of cells harboring drug-resistant BCR-ABL mutations. In vivo, however, the level of most mutations is fluctuating individually, suggesting two different clones instead of 1 compound clone containing 2 mutations.

In chronic-phase CML patients after dasatinib therapy, among 1043 patients analyzed, 174 had a mutational assessment at the time of dasatinib discontinuation.[63] In these 174 patients, 54 new mutations occurred in 47 patients (7 patients developed more than one new mutation, and 42 patients had new mutations with an IC_{50} to dasatinib >3 nM). Mutations at the time of dasatinib resistance were more common in patients with versus without mutations at the time of resistance to imatinib (see **Table 3**). The expansion of a mutant Ph+ clone initially responding to a second-generation tyrosine kinase inhibitor may be either due to late acquisition of a second mutation in the originally mutated clone, such as the T315I, or to acquisition of a completely new mutant clone, such as F317L.[64]

Sixty-four of 281 chronic-phase CML patients experienced progression during nilotinib treatment.[65] Twenty-five patients (39%) had newly detectable mutations with an IC_{50} to nilotinib greater than 150 nM, and 20 patients (31%) were bearing the same mutation as at baseline. Twenty of the 25 patients who progressed with newly detectable mutations had baseline mutations before nilotinib therapy. Thus similar to dasatinib, mutations at the time of nilotinib resistance were more common in patients with versus without mutations at the time of resistance to imatinib. The most common mutations associated with nilotinib progression were the E255K/V, F359C/V, Y253H, and T315I mutations (see **Table 3**).

SUMMARY

The most common cause of secondary imatinib resistance is point mutations in BCR-ABL that prevent effective binding of imatinib but may retain kinase activity. Over 100 point mutations coding for single amino acid substitutions in the BCR-ABL kinase domain have been isolated from imatinib resistant CML patients. Most reported mutants are rare, whereas seven mutated sites comprise two-thirds of all mutations detected. BCR-ABL mutations associated with a high degree of imatinib resistance include Y253F/H, E255K/V, H396P/R, and T315I. T315I also confers resistance to second-generation tyrosine kinase inhibitors. The early detection of BCR-ABL mutants during therapy may aid in risk stratification as well as molecular-based treatment decisions. However, the prognostic impact of BCR-ABL mutations is difficult to determine, and routine mutational analysis is not currently recommended in the absence of molecular, cytogenetic or clinical progression.

REFERENCES

1. Schindler T, Bornmann W, Pellicena P, et al. Structural mechanism for STI-571 inhibition of abelson tyrosine kinase. Science 2000;289:1938–42.
2. Corbin AS, Buchdunger E, Pascal F, et al. Analysis of the structural basis of specificity of inhibition of the ABL kinase by STI571. J Biol Chem 2002;277:32214–9.

3. Gorre ME, Mohammed M, Ellwood K, et al. Clinical resistance to STI-571 cancer therapy caused by BCR-ABL gene mutation or amplification. Science 2001;293: 876–80.
4. Hochhaus A, Kreil S, Corbin A, et al. Roots of clinical resistance to STI-571 cancer therapy. Science 2001;293:2163.
5. Barthe C, Cony-Makhoul P, Melo JV, et al. Roots of clinical resistance to STI-571 cancer therapy. Science 2001;293:2163.
6. Hochhaus A, Kreil S, Corbin AS, et al. Molecular and chromosomal mechanisms of resistance to imatinib (STI571) therapy. Leukemia 2002;16:2190–6.
7. Azam M, Latek RR, Daley GQ. Mechanisms of autoinhibition and STI-571/imatinib resistance revealed by mutagenesis of BCR-ABL. Cell 2003;112:831–43.
8. Corbin AS, La Rosée P, Stoffregen EP, et al. Several BCR-ABL kinase domain mutants associated with imatinib mesylate resistance remain sensitive to imatinib. Blood 2003;101:4611–4.
9. Shah NP, Nicoll JM, Nagar B, et al. Multiple BCR-ABL kinase domain mutations confer polyclonal resistance to the tyrosine kinase inhibitor imatinib (STI571) in chronic phase and blast crisis chronic myeloid leukemia. Cancer Cell 2002;2: 117–25.
10. Branford S, Rudzki Z, Walsh S, et al. High frequency of point mutations clustered within the adenosine triphosphate-binding region of BCR/ABL in patients with chronic myeloid leukemia or Ph-positive acute lymphoblastic leukemia who develop imatinib (STI571) resistance. Blood 2002;99:3472–5.
11. Sorel N, Chazelas F, Brizard A, et al. Double-gradient-denaturing-gradient gel electrophoresis for mutation screening of the BCR-ABL tyrosine kinase domain in chronic myeloid leukemia patients. Clin Chem 2005;51:1263–6.
12. Khorashad JS, Anand M, Marin D, et al. The presence of a BCR-ABL mutant allele in CML does not always explain clinical resistance to imatinib. Leukemia 2006;20: 658–63.
13. Poláková KM, Lopotová T, Klamová H, et al. High-resolution melt curve analysis: initial screening for mutations in BCR-ABL kinase domain. Leuk Res 2008;32: 1236–43.
14. Vivante A, Amariglio N, Koren-Michowitz M, et al. High-throughput, sensitive and quantitative assay for the detection of BCR-ABL kinase domain mutations. Leukemia 2007;21:1318–21.
15. Oehler VG, Qin J, Ramakrishnan R, et al. Absolute quantitative detection of ABL tyrosine kinase domain point mutations in chronic myeloid leukemia using a novel nanofluidic platform and mutation-specific PCR. Leukemia 2009;23: 396–9.
16. Kreuzer KA, Le Coutre P, Landt O, et al. Preexistence and evolution of imatinib mesylate-resistant clones in chronic myelogenous leukemia detected by a PNA-based PCR clamping technique. Ann Hematol 2003;82:284–9.
17. Roche-Lestienne C, Soenen-Cornu V, Grardel-Duflos N, et al. Several types of mutations of the Abl gene can be found in chronic myeloid leukemia patients resistant to STI571, and they can pre-exist to the onset of treatment. Blood 2002;100:1014–8.
18. Gruber FX, Lamark T, Anonli A, et al. Selecting and deselecting imatinib-resistant clones: observations made by longitudinal, quantitative monitoring of mutated BCR-ABL. Leukemia 2005;19:2159–65.
19. Willis SG, Lange T, Demehri S, et al. High-sensitivity detection of BCR-ABL kinase domain mutations in imatinib-naive patients: correlation with clonal cytogenetic evolution but not response to therapy. Blood 2005;106:2128–37.

20. Pelz-Ackermann O, Cross M, Pfeifer H, et al. Highly sensitive and quantitative detection of BCR-ABL kinase domain mutations by ligation PCR. Leukemia 2008;22:2288–91.

21. Preuner S, Denk D, Frommlet F, et al. Quantitative monitoring of cell clones carrying point mutations in the BCR-ABL tyrosine kinase domain by ligation-dependent polymerase chain reaction (LD-PCR). Leukemia 2008;22:1956–61.

22. Deininger MW, McGreevey L, Willis S, et al. Detection of ABL kinase domain mutations with denaturing high-performance liquid chromatography. Leukemia 2004;18:864–71.

23. Soverini S, Martinelli G, Amabile M, et al. Denaturing-HPLC-based assay for detection of ABL mutations in chronic myeloid leukemia patients resistant to Imatinib. Clin Chem 2004;50:1205–13.

24. Irving JA, O'Brien S, Lennard AL, et al. Use of denaturing HPLC for detection of mutations in the BCR-ABL kinase domain in patients resistant to Imatinib. Clin Chem 2004;50:1233–7.

25. Ernst T, Erben P, Müller MC, et al. Dynamics of BCR-ABL mutated clones prior to hematologic or cytogenetic resistance to imatinib. Haematologica 2008;93: 186–92.

26. Ernst T, Gruber FX, Pelz-Ackermann O, et al. A co-operative evaluation of different methods of detecting BCR-ABL kinase domain mutations in patients with chronic myeloid leukemia on second-line dasatinib or nilotinib therapy after failure of imatinib. Haematologica 2009;94:1227–35.

27. Apperley JF. Part I: mechanisms of resistance to imatinib in chronic myeloid leukaemia. Lancet Oncol 2007;8:1018–29.

28. O'Hare T, Eide CA, Deininger MW. BCR-ABL kinase domain mutations, drug resistance, and the road to a cure for chronic myeloid leukemia. Blood 2007; 110:2242–9.

29. Griswold IJ, MacPartlin M, Bumm T, et al. Kinase domain mutants of Bcr-Abl exhibit altered transformation potency, kinase activity and substrate utilization, irrespective of sensitivity to imatinib. Mol Cell Biol 2006;26:6082–93.

30. Skaggs BJ, Gorre ME, Ryvkin A, et al. Phosphorylation of the ATP-binding loop directs oncogenicity of drug-resistant BCR-ABL mutants. Proc Natl Acad Sci U S A 2006;103:19466–71.

31. Gruber FX, Hjorth-Hansen H, Mikkola I, et al. A novel BCR-ABL splice isoform is associated with the L248V mutation in CML patients with acquired resistance to imatinib. Leukemia 2006;20:2057–60.

32. Sherbenou DW, Hantschel O, Turaga L, et al. Characterization of BCR-ABL deletion mutants from patients with chronic myeloid leukemia. Leukemia 2008;22: 1184–90.

33. Crossmann LC, O'Hare T, Lange T, et al. A single nucleotide polymorphism in the coding region of ABL and its effects on sensitivity to imatinib. Leukemia 2005;19: 1859–62.

34. Ernst T, Hoffmann J, Erben P, et al. ABL single nucleotide polymorphisms may masquerade as BCR-ABL mutations associated with resistance to tyrosine kinase inhibitors in patients with chronic myeloid leukemia. Haematologica 2008;93: 1389–93.

35. Hochhaus A. Cytogenetic and molecular mechanisms of resistance to imatinib. Semin Hematol 2003;40:69–79.

36. Branford S, Rudzki Z, Parkinson I, et al. Real-time quantitative PCR analysis can be used as a primary screen to identify patients with CML treated with imatinib who have BCR-ABL kinase domain mutations. Blood 2004;104:2926–32.

37. Soverini S, Martinelli G, Rosti G, et al. ABL mutations in late chronic phase chronic myeloid leukemia patients with up-front cytogenetic resistance to imatinib are associated with a greater likelihood of progression to blast crisis and shorter survival: a study by the GIMEMA Working Party on Chronic Myeloid Leukemia. J Clin Oncol 2005;23:4100–9.

38. Roche-Lestienne C, Preudhomme C. Mutations in the ABL kinase domain pre-exist the onset of imatinib treatment. Semin Hematol 2003;40:80–2.

39. Chu S, Xu H, Shah NP, et al. Detection of BCR-ABL kinase mutations in CD34+ cells from chronic myelogenous leukemia patients in complete cytogenetic remission on imatinib mesylate treatment. Blood 2005;105:2093–8.

40. Graham SM, Jorgensen HG, Allan E, et al. Primitive, quiescent, Philadelphia-positive stem cells from patients with chronic myeloid leukemia are insensitive to STI571 in vitro. Blood 2002;99:319–25.

41. Angstreich GR, Matsui W, Huff CA, et al. Effects of imatinib and interferon on primitive chronic myeloid leukaemia progenitors. Br J Haematol 2005;130: 373–81.

42. Branford S, Rudzki Z, Walsh S, et al. Detection of BCR-ABL mutations in patients with CML treated with imatinib is virtually always accompanied by clinical resistance, and mutations in the ATP phosphate-binding loop (P-loop) are associated with a poor prognosis. Blood 2003;102:276–83.

43. von Bubnoff N, Manley PW, Mestan J, et al. BCR-ABL resistance screening predicts a limited spectrum of point mutations to be associated with clinical resistance to the ABL kinase inhibitor nilotinib (AMN107). Blood 2006;108:1328–33.

44. Bradeen HA, Eide CA, O'Hare T, et al. Comparison of imatinib mesylate, dasatinib (BMS-354825), and nilotinib (AMN107) in an N-ethyl-N-nitrosourea (ENU)-based mutagenesis screen: high efficacy of drug combinations. Blood 2006;108: 2332–8.

45. Redaelli S, Piazza R, Rostagno R, et al. Activity of bosutinib, dasatinib, and nilotinib against 18 imatinib-resistant BCR/ABL mutants. J Clin Oncol 2009;27: 469–71.

46. Gontarewicz A, Balabanov S, Keller G, et al. Simultaneous targeting of Aurora kinases and Bcr-Abl kinase by the small molecule inhibitor PHA-739358 is effective against imatinib-resistant BCR-ABL mutations including T315I. Blood 2008; 111:4355–64.

47. Nicolini FE, Mauro MJ, Martinelli G, et al. Epidemiologic study on survival of chronic myeloid leukemia and Ph(+) acute lymphoblastic leukemia patients with BCR-ABL T315I mutation. Blood 2009;114:5271–8.

48. O'Hare T, Shakespeare WC, Zhu X, et al. AP24534, a pan-BCR-ABL inhibitor for chronic myeloid leukemia, potently inhibits the T315I mutant and overcomes mutation-based resistance. Cancer Cell 2009;16:401–12.

49. Laneuville P, Dilea C, Yin OQ, et al. Comparative in vitro cellular data alone are insufficient to predict clinical responses and guide the choice of BCR-ABL inhibitor for treating imatinib-resistant chronic myeloid leukemia. J Clin Oncol 2010;28: e169–71.

50. Khorashad JS, de Lavallade H, Apperley JF, et al. Finding of kinase domain mutations in patients with chronic phase chronic myeloid leukemia responding to imatinib may identify those at high risk of disease progression. J Clin Oncol 2008; 26:4806–13.

51. Sherbenou DW, Wong MJ, Humayun A, et al. Mutations of the BCR-ABL-kinase domain occur in a minority of patients with stable complete cytogenetic response to imatinib. Leukemia 2007;21:489–93.

52. Lange T, Park B, Willis SG, et al. BCR-ABL kinase domain mutations in chronic myeloid leukemia: not quite enough to cause resistance to imatinib therapy? Cell Cycle 2005;4:1761–6.
53. Pfeifer H, Wassmann B, Pavlova A, et al. Kinase domain mutations of BCR-ABL frequently precede imatinib-based therapy and give rise to relapse in patients with de novo Philadelphia-positive acute lymphoblastic leukemia (Ph+ ALL). Blood 2007;110:727–34.
54. Müller MC, Lahaye T, Hochhaus A. Resistance to tumor specific therapy with imatinib by clonal selection of mutated cells. Dtsch Med Wochenschr 2002;127:2205–7.
55. Hanfstein B, Mueller MC, Kreil S, et al. Dynamics of mutant BCR-ABL positive clones after cessation of imatinib treatment. Haematologica 2008;93(s1):43–4.
56. Tipping AJ, Mahon FX, Zafirides G, et al. Drug responses of imatinib mesylate-resistant cells: synergism of imatinib with other chemotherapeutic drugs. Leukemia 2002;16:2349–57.
57. Legros L, Hayette S, Nicolini FE, et al. BCR-ABL(T315I) transcript disappearance in an imatinib-resistant CML patient treated with homoharringtonine: a new therapeutic challenge? Leukemia 2007;21:2204–6.
58. Shah NP, Tran C, Lee FY, et al. Overriding imatinib resistance with a novel ABL kinase inhibitor. Science 2004;305:399–401.
59. Weisberg E, Manley PW, Breitenstein W, et al. Characterization of AMN107, a selective inhibitor of native and mutant Bcr-Abl. Cancer Cell 2005;7:129–41.
60. Burgess MR, Skaggs BJ, Shah NP, et al. Comparative analysis of two clinically active BCR-ABL kinase inhibitors reveals the role of conformation-specific binding in resistance. Proc Natl Acad Sci U S A 2005;102:3395–400.
61. Ray A, Cowan-Jacob SW, Manley PW, et al. Identification of BCR-ABL point mutations conferring resistance to the Abl kinase inhibitor AMN107 (nilotinib) by a random mutagenesis study. Blood 2007;109:5011–5.
62. Shah NP, Skaggs BJ, Branford S, et al. Sequential ABL kinase inhibitor therapy selects for compound drug-resistant BCR-ABL mutations with altered oncogenic potency. J Clin Invest 2007;117:2562–9.
63. Müller MC, Cortes JE, Kim DW, et al. Dasatinib treatment of chronic-phase chronic myeloid leukemia: analysis of responses according to preexisting BCR-ABL mutations. Blood 2009;114:4944–53.
64. Khorashad JS, Milojkovic D, Mehta P, et al. In vivo kinetics of kinase domain mutations in CML patients treated with dasatinib after failing imatinib. Blood 2008;111:2378–81.
65. Hughes T, Saglio G, Branford S, et al. Impact of baseline BCR-ABL mutations on response to nilotinib in patients with chronic myeloid leukemia in chronic phase. J Clin Oncol 2009;27:4204–10.

Selection of Therapy: Rational Decisions Based on Molecular Events

Jamshid S. Khorashad, MD, PhD[a], Michael W.N. Deininger, MD, PhD[b],*

KEYWORDS

- Chronic myeloid leukemia • Imatinib • Resistance • BCR-ABL
- Mutation • hOCT1

Chronic myeloid leukemia (CML) is a hematopoietic stem cell malignancy caused by BCR-ABL, a fusion protein derived from a reciprocal translocation between chromosomes 9 and 22 [t(9;22)(q34;q11)], cytogenetically visible as the Philadelphia chromosome. BCR-ABL is a constitutively active tyrosine kinase that activates multiple signaling pathways, thereby promoting the expansion of myeloid cells. The clinical result is a myeloproliferative neoplasm characterized by an increase of neutrophils and their precursors. In the initial chronic phase (CP) cellular differentiation is largely intact, and the disease is easily managed with drug treatment. In the absence of effective therapy, CML progresses to an acute leukemia, termed blastic phase (BP), sometimes through an intermediary state, termed accelerated phase (AP).[1] BP CML has a poor prognosis, with survival frequently measured in weeks. The realization that the kinase activity of BCR-ABL is central to CML pathogenesis led to the development of imatinib, a small-molecule adenosine triphosphate (ATP)-competitive tyrosine kinase inhibitor (TKI), as a rational molecularly targeted therapy. Subsequently the second-line TKIs, nilotinib and dasatinib, were introduced, initially for the treatment of patients who failed imatinib and recently for the treatment of newly diagnosed patients.[2] All these drugs inhibit BCR-ABL activity, thereby blocking the activation of downstream signals critical for proliferation and survival of CML cells.[3] However, they are distinct by their differential potency against the primary target, activity profiles

Funding: This study was supported by NIH grants HL082978-01 (M.W.D.) and CA04963920A2 (M.W.D.), the Leukemia and Lymphoma Society grant 7036-01 (M.W.D.). M.W.D. is a Scholar in Clinical Research of the Leukemia and Lymphoma Society.
[a] Deininger Lab, Huntsman Cancer Institute, University of Utah, 2000 Circle of Hope, Room 4270, Salt Lake City, UT 84112-5550, USA
[b] Division of Hematology and Hematologic Malignancies, Huntsman Cancer Institute, University of Utah, 2000 Circle of Hope, Room 4280, Salt Lake City, UT 84112-5550, USA
* Corresponding author.
E-mail address: michael.deininger@hci.utah.edu

Hematol Oncol Clin N Am 25 (2011) 1009–1023
doi:10.1016/j.hoc.2011.09.006
0889-8588/11/$ – see front matter Published by Elsevier Inc.

hemonc.theclinics.com

against BCR-ABL mutants, and "off-target" effects against kinases other than BCR-ABL. Third-generation TKIs, such as ponatinib and DC-2036, are in clinical development and will add additional diversity to the therapeutic space.

In this article the authors review to what extent molecular data can be used to rationalize therapeutic choices. This discussion includes two categories of data: first, markers that globally measure risk, but do not provide a molecular rationale for therapy selection; and second, biomarkers with a causal link to a clinical phenotype, such as certain mutations of the BCR-ABL kinase domain. Despite considerable progress on both fronts, as of 2011 therapy selection is still mainly based on clinical criteria, therefore the authors have decided to discuss molecular biomarkers in the context of available clinical prognostication tools. Given the extensive literature on the prognostic value of BCR-ABL transcripts and their dynamics during therapy, this article focuses on biomarkers that do not directly reflect disease burden as a surrogate of responsiveness to treatment, and the reader is referred to excellent reviews of this topic.[4]

RISK STRATIFICATION
Disease Phase

The most important clinical tool in risk-stratifying CML patients is the phase of disease. Irrespective of the type of therapy, results tend to be best in CP, intermediate in AP, and poor in BP. The early studies of imatinib in patients who had failed prior interferon-α (IFN)-based therapies impressively confirmed the previous experience with IFN, conventional cytotoxic agents such as hydrea, and allogeneic stem cell transplant. Results from the International Randomized Study of Interferon and STI571 (IRIS) and other single-center or community-based studies uniformly show that imatinib is most effective in early CP, with higher rates of complete cytogenetic response (CCyR) and major molecular response (MMR) in newly diagnosed patients in comparison with patients treated in late CP, defined as treatment initiation later than 1 year from diagnosis or after failure of IFN (**Table 1**).[5–7] Response rates and the durability of responses are much lower in the AP/BP than in the CP (early or late).[8–12] Compared with imatinib, nilotinib and dasatinib were shown to result in higher rates of CCyR and MMR in newly diagnosed patients[13–17]; however, similar to imatinib, response rates and durability were lower in the patients treated in late CP, AP, or BP.[18,19] There are two major messages from these data. First, the fact that none of the approved TKIs are able to completely abolish the effects of longer disease duration or progression suggests that the mechanisms underlying failure overlap; second, the fact that patient populations that meet the criteria for CP have very different response rates is evidence that CP defined on clinical/morphologic grounds must encompass a spectrum of disorders. Compared with CP, AP is even more heterogeneous and represents the most difficult category in terms of outcome prediction. As few data are available on the results of TKI therapy in patients who are diagnosed in AP, it is likely that this uncommon group will encompass some patients who are biologically in CP. From

Table 1 Response to imatinib according to disease phase			
Disease Phase		**CCyR (%)**	**Overall Survival (%)**
Chronic phase (CP)	Newly diagnosed[7,21]	5 years ~78–82	5 years ~83–89
	Late CP[6]	5 years ~55	5 years ~77
Accelerated phase[8,10]		~17	12 months ~74
Blastic phase[11,12]		~7	12 months ~32

the perspective of the developed world, where some 90% of patients are diagnosed in CP, the most important question is whether one can accurately identify high-risk patients who are in CP by morphologic criteria.

Clinical Risk Stratification in CP

The first clinical risk-stratification tool for newly diagnosed CP patients was established by Sokal and colleagues[20] in a cohort of patients treated with cytotoxic drugs. Age, spleen size, platelet count, and the percentage of blast cells in the peripheral blood were identified as independent variables in multivariate analysis.[20] Remarkably, the predictive value of the Sokal score was subsequently confirmed in patients treated with IFN, imatinib, and nilotinib.[7,14,21,22] That the Sokal score is predictive of response irrespective of therapy suggests that it identifies critical biological disease features. Whether this reflects a biological quality that is present ab initio or acquired during a preceding period of undiagnosed disease is unknown. Subsequent studies were aimed at improving the Sokal score. By including more parameters in the multivariate analysis, Hasford and colleagues[23] developed a new score (Euro score) comprising blood eosinophil and basophil counts in addition to the factors used in the Sokal score. The Euro score was superior in predicting survival in patients treated with IFN patients. Recently, a new prognostic score (EUTOS; European Treatment and Outcome Study for CML) was reported for patients treated with imatinib. The EUTOS score is based only on the percentage of basophils in blood and on spleen size, and was shown to be superior to both the Sokal and the Euro scores in its prognostic ability.[24]

The Hammersmith group developed a score for early identification of responders to the second-line TKIs nilotinib and dasatinib.[25,26] This prognostication system is based on 3 factors: previous cytogenetic response to imatinib; Sokal risk at diagnosis; and recurrent neutropenia during imatinib therapy.[25] Other groups reported that patients with poor performance status and no previous cytogenetic response to imatinib therapy had a low likelihood of responding to second-generation TKIs and should be offered additional treatment options.[27,28] These observations suggest that in vivo drug sensitivity, that is, the response to initial therapy (ie, a cytogenetic response) identifies a good risk group of patients, and that this good risk is to some extent carried over to salvage therapies. This proposal is consistent with experience in oncology, where failure after an initial response is usually prognostically more favorable than a primary refractory disease.

Cytogenetic clonal evolution (CE) refers to the presence or development of karyotypic abnormalities in addition to the Philadelphia chromosome (**Table 2**). In some studies its presence at diagnosis was associated with poor prognosis.[29,30] In the pre-IFN era, CE was noted in 30% to 50% of the patients before blastic transformation, and was considered as diagnostic of an accelerated phase.[31,32] However, some patients who developed cytogenetic CE on IFN therapy continued in CP for long periods, with the occasional disappearance of CE.[33] In patients treated with imatinib in late CP after IFN failure, CE was not a significant prognostic factor for major cytogenetic response.[34] Subsequent studies confirmed this initial finding, but identified CE as an independently poor prognostic factor for survival and relapse-free survival in CP and AP CML.[35,36] Why CE appears to affect overall and relapse-free survival, but not cytogenetic response, remains unexplained. CE was also shown to be associated with detection of low-level BCR-ABL kinase domain (KD) mutations in imatinib-naïve patients, suggesting that both may reflect underlying genetic instability.[37] While at present the prognostic significance of CE at the time of diagnosis remains somewhat controversial, there is consensus that acquisition of CE after start of imatinib indicates such a high risk of relapse that it is now considered failure.[38–40]

Table 2
Common additional cytogenetic abnormalities in Philadelphia chromosome–positive cells

Abnormality	% of Cases with Additional Cytogenetic Changes
Trisomy 8	34
Second Philadelphia chromosome	30
Isochromosome 17	20
Trisomy 19	13
Loss of the Y chromosome	8 (of males)
Trisomy 21	7
Trisomy 17	5
Monosomy 7	5

Data from Mitelman F. The cytogenetic scenario of chronic myeloid leukemia. Leuk Lymphoma 1993;11 Suppl 1:11–5; and Johansson B, Fioretos T, Mitelman F. Cytogenetic and molecular genetic evolution of chronic myeloid leukemia. Acta Haematol 2002;107:76–94.

Limited data are available in patients treated with second-line TKIs, but results are generally similar. Of note, the impact of specific abnormalities is variable: trisomy 8, chromosome 17, and complex abnormalities are associated with the worst outcome.[41]

While the established risk scores based on standard diagnostic tests provide some information on the risk of CP patients, they are too imprecise to inform far-reaching clinical decisions. In addition, they are mostly epiphenomenal and do not identify the molecular causes underlying the higher risk of treatment failure or progression to advanced phase. To overcome this shortcoming genome-wide approaches as well as functional assays have been explored to develop more precise prediction tools.

Genome-Wide Scanning

Several groups have embarked on genome-wide scanning approaches to identify biomarkers that predict CP response to TKI therapy. Various technology platforms have been used, including gene-expression profiling and array comparative genomic hybridization (CGH). In a retrospective study of patients treated with chemotherapy (mostly hydroxyurea), Yong and colleagues[42] investigated the gene expression profile of CD34$^+$ cells stored at diagnosis and identified several genes (CD7, proteinase 3, elastase) whose level of expression was correlated with the duration of CP. Radich and colleagues[43] compared gene expression in CP, AP, and BP bone marrow cells and observed phase-specific expression patterns that distinguished between CP and AP/BP. By contrast, expression patterns in AP and BP were very similar, suggesting that CML is essentially a 2-phase rather than 3-phase disease. These investigators also saw significant overlap between the gene-expression patterns of patients with resistance to imatinib with that of patients in AP/BP, and found that samples from patients in second CP after blastic transformation had essentially maintained the profile of BP, indicating that a morphologic remission fails to turn back the "biological clock" of the disease. In aggregate these findings indicate that the biological features of imatinib resistance and disease progression overlap and override morphologic criteria. This notion was further supported by an independent study by McWeeney and colleagues,[44] who studied the gene expression profiles of CD34$^+$ cells from patients in CP prior to imatinib treatment and identified a gene expression classifier that correlated with subsequent cytogenetic response. In meta-analysis they detected overlap between the expression profiles of imatinib nonresponders with those of short CP in the study by Yong and colleagues,[42] and BP in another study that compared gene expression profiles in CD34$^+$ cells from patients with CP versus myeloid BP, further supporting the association between TKI failure and progression to AP/BC.[45,46] It is likely that not all of these prognostically important genes directly confer resistance. For example, myeloid differentiation genes such as ELA2, MPO, CSTA, CSTG, and PRTN3 are downregulated in prospective nonresponders (McWeeney and colleagues) and patients with a short CP (Yong and colleagues), an expression pattern consistent with the differentiation block that characterizes transformation from CP to AP/BP. Whether this differentiation block itself is causal to resistance remains to be established. From the point of clinical utility it is desirable to limit the number of genes necessary to predict molecularly advanced disease. Toward this goal the Seattle group recently reported a refinement of their molecular prediction algorithm to a set of only 6 genes (NOB1, DDX47, IGSF2, LTB4R, SCARB1, and SLC25A3) that distinguish between CP and AP/BP.[47] Validation of these data in independent studies will be required before this classifier is used clinically. CGH or single-nucleotide polymorphism arrays were used to investigate genomic aberrations at the DNA level in newly diagnosed patients and during the progression of disease from CP to BC.[48–50] Recurrent cryptic losses on certain chromosomes in CML CD34$^+$ cells were correlated with loss of response to imatinib.[51] Perhaps because of rather small sample sizes and the heterogeneity among the various studies, no consistent pattern has emerged as yet, and additional validation studies will be required.[51–54]

MEASURING SENSITIVITY TO BCR-ABL INHIBITORS

A different approach to response prediction would be to establish correlations between target inhibition and clinical response. Several groups reported that the extent of in vitro inhibition of BCR-ABL by imatinib in primary cells from newly diagnosed CML patients is correlated with subsequent clinical response,[55–58] whereas another study did not find such a correlation.[59] The conflicting results could be attributable to the technical differences such as the source of investigated cells (fresh or cryopreserved CD34$^+$ cells), different culture conditions, and differences in drug concentrations and exposure times to imatinib. Another approach is to quantify the in vivo BCR-ABL kinase inhibition in the first month of imatinib therapy. In a prospective study the degree of BCR-ABL inhibition (measured using immunoblots to quantify CrkL phosphorylation as a surrogate marker) was shown to be an excellent predictor of cytogenetic and molecular response.[60] As this study was based on analysis of mononuclear cells (MNC) at different time points following treatment initiation, it is possible that the reduced kinase activity reflected a relative reduction of leukemic cells rather than the inhibition of kinase activity. Another approach to predict in vivo sensitivity is to measure the TKI inhibition of primary cells cultured ex vivo. For example, there is a fairly good correlation between imatinib inhibition of colony formation and clinical response.[61] Unfortunately, all of these assays are too cumbersome for routine purposes.

DRUG TRANSPORTERS

Imatinib is subject to active transport mechanisms, and the expression of several drug transporters has been shown to correlate with response, although some of the data remain controversial. For example, while in vitro studies in cell lines have demonstrated that imatinib, nilotinib, and dasatinib are all substrates of the ABCB1 and

ABCG2 ion transporters, there is little evidence that these mechanisms are operational in primary CML progenitor cells.[62–65] By contrast, there is a fairly large body of data supporting the role of hOCT1 in active transport of imatinib into the cells and in association with response to imatinib therapy.[66,67] For example, White and colleagues[68,69] reported that higher hOCT1 activity at diagnosis in MNC was predictive of optimal long-term outcome in CML patients treated with imatinib in CP. Unexpectedly, hOCT1 seems to be more important for imatinib transport in differentiated cells as compared with CD34$^+$ cells, where expression is low and not predictive of response.[63] The reason for these counterintuitive observations remains unclear, but it is likely that some of the discrepancies in the published data reflect differences in the composition of the cells analyzed in the various studies.[70] Another problem is the use of prazosin to block the hOCT1 channel for measurement of hOCT1 activity. Because prazosin may target other transporters, this assay could overemphasize the role of hOCT1 as the main transporter of imatinib. Consistent with this, in vitro studies found that imatinib is a poor substrate for hOCT1 and concluded that this transporter is unlikely to contribute substantially to the deposition and activity profile of imatinib. Nevertheless, prazosin sensitivity might provide a composite surrogate for the activity of several transporters that are relevant to the intracellular uptake and retention of imatinib.[71] In addition to hOCT1 activity,[69] high hOCT1 expression was also shown to predict response to imatinib.[67,72,73] As of now hOCT1 activity is one of the few biomarkers that might indeed influence therapeutic decisions, because higher doses of imatinib (600 mg/d) have been shown to overcome the negative effect of low hOCT1 activity on response.[69] Unfortunately, the predictive value of hOCT1 remains limited to imatinib, as the active transport of imatinib through hOCT1 does not seem to have any role in transport of nilotinib or dasatinib.[74,75]

MOLECULAR MARKERS IN SECOND-LINE THERAPY

It is estimated that approximately 20% to 40% of newly diagnosed CP patients will eventually require switching to dasatinib or nilotinib for intolerance or resistance.[40,70,76–79] Although the mechanisms governing primary resistance remain poorly understood, many patients with acquired imatinib resistance have missense mutations in the BCR-ABL KD that reduce TKI sensitivity to various degrees depending on the mutation type and specific TKI.[80–84] Given that dasatinib and nilotinib may eventually replace imatinib in front-line therapy, the mutation spectrum in second-line therapy will change dramatically.[13,14] T315I was the first BCR-ABL KD mutation detected in clinical samples,[85] and is the only mutant resistant to imatinib and both second-line TKIs dasatinib and nilotinib.[86] Many other mutants detected in clinical samples have been validated biochemically and exhibit various degrees of resistance to available TKIs, supporting clinical decisions in a subset of patients.

KD Mutations in Imatinib-Naïve Patients

Several studies have analyzed KD mutations in pre-imatinib samples using highly sensitive techniques. However, there was no apparent correlation between the presence of mutations and response; if resistance developed the mutation initially present was not necessarily present at the time of relapse. Therefore there is no role for the detection of mutations at a very low level before treatment. Whether patients with advanced disease should be screened is a matter of debate; because most of these patients will have received TKI therapy, and this will usually be part of a resistance workup.[37,87–89] Of importance is that the situation in CML is different from Philadelphia chromosome–positive acute lymphoblastic leukemia (ALL), where BCR-ABL KD mutations conferring high-level imatinib resistance are present in a substantial proportion of patients at diagnosis, and eventually give rise to relapse.[90]

BCR-ABL KD Mutations in Patients on Imatinib

Mutations not only cause resistance to imatinib and loss of response, but are also shown to be associated with outcome, irrespective of their level of TKI resistance. Specifically, several studies showed that mutations of the ATP-binding loop (p-loop) were associated with poor prognosis in patients on imatinib.[83,91] One possible explanation for the poor clinical outcome of patients with p-loop mutation could be the increased transformation potency of p-loop mutants Y253F and E255K observed in the in vitro experiments.[92] Less surprisingly, other studies found correlations between the level of imatinib resistance and outcome, reflecting the efficacy of available treatment.[93] It is obvious that such correlations are valid only in the context of a specific TKI, with a specific activity profile.

The detection of mutations in patients who are responding to imatinib therapy is considered a "warning sign," as it is associated with a higher risk of loss of response.[93,94] For example, in a study of patients who had achieved CCyR, the detection of a KD mutation was the only significant predictor for loss of CCyR.[93] Of interest, the detection of KD mutation at the time of resistance to imatinib predicts a higher likelihood of developing other KD mutations after starting second-line TKIs.[88,95] Higher genetic instability might be responsible for the "development" of the secondary mutations, which may have existed before the start of salvage therapy, but were suppressed to low levels by the dominant mutant clone. Together these data suggest that KD mutations measure several different parameters influencing outcome: those related to biochemical consequences at the target level (high vs low level resistance mutations; hypomorphic or hypermorphic kinase alleles with increased or reduced transforming potency[92,96]) and others that provide an indirect measurement of critical disease features, such as genomic instability.

KD Mutations and Selection of Second-Line Therapy

In vitro studies have provided information about the sensitivity of the different BCR-ABL KD mutants to second-line TKIs, which provides guidance for choosing the appropriate drug after imatinib failure.[80,81] A study by the Adelaide group suggested that screening for KD mutations may provide useful clinical information in some 43% of cases.[97] However, the clinical sensitivity of the various mutants to the second-line TKIs does not completely match the in vitro predictions. For example, the Y253H, E255K, and F359V/C mutants are sensitive to nilotinib in vitro, but largely resistant in clinical studies. Similarly, F317L and V299L are moderately resistant to dasatinib in vitro, but highly resistant in vivo (**Table 3**). Thus the use of in vitro data alone to guide the choice of TKI for patients can be misleading, as this does not take into account important in vivo variables such as protein binding and cell influx/efflux.[98] The exception is the T315I mutation, which consistently confers resistance to all currently approved TKIs.[97] With this in mind, the most important information from mutational analysis of the BCR-ABL KD is whether T315I is present or not. Several studies showed that the impact of T315I on survival depended on the disease phase at the time of detection, suggesting that while T315I is a highly resistant mutant, it is not by itself associated with a more aggressive biological phenotype.[99] In support of this, T315I was shown to exhibit reduced kinase activity in vitro.[94] Although it remains somewhat controversial as to whether T315I is indeed a loss-of-function mutant,[92,100] it can explain why the mutant clone can regress after discontinuation of therapy.[101,102] Patients with a T315I mutation will not benefit from dasatinib or

Table 3
Sensitivity of mutants to nilotinib and dasatinib

Nilotinib			Dasatinib		
In vitro		In vivo	In vitro		In vivo
O'Hare et al[81]	Redaelli et al[80]	Branford et al[97]	O'Hare et al[81]	Radaelli et al[80]	Branford et al[97]
T315I[a]	T315I[a]	T315I	T315I/A[a]	T315I[a]	T315I/A
Y253H[b]	E255V[a]	Y253H	F317L[b]	V299L[c]	V299L
E255V[b]	E255K[c]	E255K/V	V299L[b]	E255K[c]	F317L/I/C/V
E255K[b]	F359V[c]	F359V/C	E255V[b]	L248V[c]	
F359V[b]	G250E[c]		F317L[b]	F317L[c]	
Y253F[b]	Y253F[b]		E255K[b]	G250E[c]	
Q252H[b]	H396R[b]		Q252H[b]	E255V[b]	
T315A[b]	L248V[b]			Q252H[b]	
V379I[b]	Q252H[b]			F486S[b]	
	H396P[b]			L384M[b]	
	L384M[b]				
	F317L[b]				
	E279K[b]				

[a] Highly resistant according to in vitro studies.
[b] Moderately resistant/sensitive according to in vitro studies.
[c] Resistant according to in vitro studies.
Data from Branford S, Melo JV, Hughes TP. Selecting optimal second-line tyrosine kinase inhibitor therapy for chronic myeloid leukemia patients after imatinib failure—does the BCRABL mutation status really matter? Blood 2009;114(27):5426–35.

nilotinib, and should be offered an experimental drug if they are in CP and allogeneic stem cell transplantation if they have progressed to AP/BP. The most promising experimental agent is ponatinib, a multitargeted kinase inhibitor that is active against all BCR-ABL mutants tested, including T315I. In vitro mutagenesis screens failed to reveal any new single mutation liability, in contrast to second-line TKIs tested with the same experimental system.[103] Results from a phase 1 study have shown considerable activity in CP patients who failed 2 or more TKIs, including imatinib. It is interesting that the rate of CCyR was higher in patients with T315I than in patients with other KD mutations or without mutations.[104] Thus, effective treatment can turn a poor prognostic marker into a favorable one. A speculative explanation for this is that CML that escapes from TKI therapy through acquisition of T315I identifies itself as extremely dependent on BCR-ABL and, as such, extremely sensitive to restoration of BCR-ABL inhibition with ponatinib.

Prognostic Biomarkers or Scores at the Start of Second-Line TKI

While the type of KD mutation is a valuable molecular marker in predicting response to second-line TKIs, many patients do not have mutations, and the correlation with response/resistance is tight only toward the "negative" side (T315I). However, other biomarkers may be able to capture the underlying risk biology. For example *EVI-1* expression at the point of imatinib failure has been shown to identify patients who are likely to fail on second-line regimens, and might be better served by early referral for allogeneic transplantation.[105] As discussed earlier, BCR-ABL KD mutations predict a higher risk of developing (or: unmasking) secondary mutations on second-line TKI therapy.[88,95] Further investigations are needed to provide information on what pattern of gene expression or molecular markers can be used as prognostic tools for patients who start dasatinib or nilotinib as the first line of therapy or after imatinib failure.

FUTURE DIRECTIONS

An honest account of molecular biomarkers in CML is that the only tool with broad clinical impact in 2011 is screening for KD mutations. All other prognostication relies on routine clinical and laboratory measurements that define disease stage and conventional risk scores. One could even argue that biomarkers in CML will never see their prime time, given the high rates of CCyR and low risk of progression in newly diagnosed patients treated with second-generation TKIs.[13,14] However, this is an unlikely scenario for two reasons,. First, imatinib will come off patent in 2015, and the question will arise whether we can identify a patient population that will do equally well with a generic drug that will be far less expensive than second-generation TKIs. In an era of runaway health care costs, this will have major health-economic implications. Prospective studies will be critical to support a biomarker-based approach to initial therapy. Second, therapeutic goals will shift toward disease eradication, and the ability of TKIs to annihilate the leukemic cell clone may be correlated with molecular disease features present at diagnosis. In support of this, a high Sokal risk score was highly predictive of disease recurrence in the Stop Imatinib (STIM) trial, where patients with a complete molecular response to imatinib discontinued therapy.[106] Thus, there may be 3 categories of CP patients at diagnosis: a first group, probably a small minority, who will achieve sustained molecular negativity and can eventually discontinue therapy; a second group, for whom this may be achieved by combining TKIs with another biochemical therapeutic modality; and a third group, for whom only an immunologic approach such as allogeneic transplant is capable of permanently suppressing or even eradicating the CML clone. To maximize the impact of biomarker studies, undoubtedly it will be important not only to develop molecular markers but also to convert this knowledge into novel and rational targeted therapies. We still have a long way to go, but the first steps have been taken.

ACKNOWLEDGMENTS

The authors thank Suzanne Wickens for administrative support.

REFERENCES

1. Goldman JM, Melo JV. Chronic myeloid leukemia—advances in biology and new approaches to treatment. N Engl J Med 2003;349:1451–64.
2. Giles FJ, Rosti G, Beris P, et al. Nilotinib is superior to imatinib as first-line therapy of chronic myeloid leukemia: the ENESTnd study. Expert Rev Hematol 2010;3:665–73.
3. Deininger M, Buchdunger E, Druker BJ. The development of imatinib as a therapeutic agent for chronic myeloid leukemia. Blood 2005;105:2640–53.
4. Hughes TP, Hochhaus A, Branford S, et al. Long-term prognostic significance of early molecular response to imatinib in newly diagnosed chronic myeloid leukemia: an analysis from the International Randomized Study of Interferon and STI571 (IRIS). Blood 2010;116:3758–65.
5. Scerni AC, Alvares LA, Beltrao AC, et al. Influence of late treatment on how chronic myeloid leukemia responds to imatinib. Clinics (Sao Paulo) 2009;64:731–4.
6. Palandri F, Iacobucci I, Martinelli G, et al. Long-term outcome of complete cytogenetic responders after imatinib 400 mg in late chronic phase, Philadelphia-positive chronic myeloid leukemia: the GIMEMA Working Party on CML. J Clin Oncol 2008;26:106–11.

7. Druker B, Guilhot F, O'Brien S, et al. Five-year follow-up of imatinib therapy for newly diagnosed chronic myelogenous leukemia in chronic-phase shows sustained responses and high overall survival. N Engl J Med 2006;355:2408–17.
8. Cortes J, Kantarjian H. Advanced-phase chronic myeloid leukemia. Semin Hematol 2003;40:79–86.
9. Goldman JM, Marin D, Olavarria E, et al. Clinical decisions for chronic myeloid leukemia in the imatinib era. Semin Hematol 2003;40:98–103.
10. Talpaz M, Silver RT, Druker BJ, et al. Imatinib induces durable hematologic and cytogenetic responses in patients with accelerated phase chronic myeloid leukemia: results of a phase 2 study. Blood 2002;99:1928–37.
11. Sawyers CL, Hochhaus A, Feldman E, et al. Imatinib induces hematologic and cytogenetic responses in patients with chronic myelogenous leukemia in myeloid blast crisis: results of a phase II study. Blood 2002;99:3530–9.
12. Kantarjian HM, Cortes J, O'Brien S, et al. Imatinib mesylate (STI571) therapy for Philadelphia chromosome-positive chronic myelogenous leukemia in blast phase. Blood 2002;99:3547–53.
13. Kantarjian H, Shah NP, Hochhaus A, et al. Dasatinib versus imatinib in newly diagnosed chronic-phase chronic myeloid leukemia. N Engl J Med 2010;362: 2260–70.
14. Saglio G, Kim DW, Issaragrisil S, et al. Nilotinib versus imatinib for newly diagnosed chronic myeloid leukemia. N Engl J Med 2010;362:2251–9.
15. Giles FJ, Abruzzese E, Rosti G, et al. Nilotinib is active in chronic and accelerated phase chronic myeloid leukemia following failure of imatinib and dasatinib therapy. Leukemia 2010;24:1299–301.
16. Apperley JF, Cortes JE, Kim DW, et al. Dasatinib in the treatment of chronic myeloid leukemia in accelerated phase after imatinib failure: the START a trial. J Clin Oncol 2009;27:3472–9.
17. Saglio G, Hochhaus A, Goh YT, et al. Dasatinib in imatinib-resistant or imatinib-intolerant chronic myeloid leukemia in blast phase after 2 years of follow-up in a phase 3 study: efficacy and tolerability of 140 milligrams once daily and 70 milligrams twice daily. Cancer 2010;116:3852–61.
18. Kantarjian HM, Giles F, Gattermann N, et al. Nilotinib (formerly AMN107), a highly selective Bcr-Abl tyrosine kinase inhibitor, is effective in patients with Philadelphia chromosome-positive chronic myelogenous leukemia in chronic phase following imatinib resistance and intolerance. Blood 2007;110:3540–6.
19. Cortes J, Rousselot P, Kim DW, et al. Dasatinib induces complete hematologic and cytogenetic responses in patients with imatinib-resistant or -intolerant chronic myeloid leukemia in blast crisis. Blood 2007;109:3207–13.
20. Sokal JE, Cox EB, Baccarani M, et al. Prognostic discrimination in "good-risk" chronic granulocytic leukemia. Blood 1984;63:789–99.
21. de Lavallade H, Apperley JF, Khorashad JS, et al. Imatinib for newly diagnosed patients with chronic myeloid leukaemia: incidence of sustained responses in an intention-to-treat analysis. J Clin Oncol 2008;26:3358–63.
22. Hehlmann R, Ansari H, Hasford J, et al. Comparative analysis of the impact of risk profile and of drug therapy on survival in CML using Sokal's index and a new score. German chronic myeloid leukaemia (CML)-Study Group. Br J Haematol 1997;97:76–85.
23. Hasford J, Pfirrmann M, Hehlmann R, et al. A new prognostic score for survival of patients with chronic myeloid leukemia treated with interferon alfa. Writing Committee for the Collaborative CML Prognostic Factors Project Group. J Natl Cancer Inst 1998;90:850–8.

24. Hasford J, Baccarani M, Hoffmann V, et al. Predicting complete cytogenetic response and subsequent progression-free survival in 2060 patients with CML on imatinib treatment: the EUTOS score. Blood 2011;118(3):686–92.
25. Milojkovic D, Nicholson E, Apperley JF, et al. Early prediction of success or failure of treatment with second-generation tyrosine kinase inhibitors in patients with chronic myeloid leukemia. Haematologica 2010;95:224–31.
26. Breccia M, Stagno F, Gozzini A, et al. Hammersmith score application identifies chronic myeloid leukemia patients with poor prognosis before treatment with second-generation tyrosine kinase inhibitors. Am J Hematol 2011;86:523–5.
27. Jabbour E, Kantarjian H, O'Brien S, et al. Predictive factors for outcome and response in patients treated with second-generation tyrosine kinase inhibitors for chronic myeloid leukemia in chronic phase after imatinib failure. Blood 2011;117:1822–7.
28. Tam CS, Kantarjian H, Garcia-Manero G, et al. Failure to achieve a major cytogenetic response by twelve months defines inadequate response in patients receiving nilotinib or dasatinib as second or subsequent line therapy for chronic myeloid leukemia. Blood 2008;112:516–8.
29. Kantarjian HM, Smith TL, McCredie KB, et al. Chronic myelogenous leukemia: a multivariate analysis of the associations of patient characteristics and therapy with survival. Blood 1985;66:1326–35.
30. Sokal JE, Gomez GA, Baccarani M, et al. Prognostic significance of additional cytogenetic abnormalities at diagnosis of Philadelphia chromosome-positive chronic granulocytic leukemia. Blood 1988;72:294–8.
31. Kantarjian HM, Dixon D, Keating MJ, et al. Characteristics of accelerated disease in chronic myelogenous leukemia. Cancer 1988;61:1441–6.
32. Sessarego M, Panarello C, Coviello DA, et al. Karyotype evolution in CML: high frequency of translocations other than the Ph. Cancer Genet Cytogenet 1987; 25:73–80.
33. Majlis A, Smith TL, Talpaz M, et al. Significance of cytogenetic clonal evolution in chronic myelogenous leukemia. J Clin Oncol 1996;14:196–203.
34. Kantarjian H, Sawyers C, Hochhaus A, et al. Hematologic and cytogenetic responses to imatinib mesylate in chronic myelogenous leukemia. N Engl J Med 2002;346:645–52.
35. Cortes JE, Talpaz M, Giles F, et al. Prognostic significance of cytogenetic clonal evolution in patients with chronic myelogenous leukemia on imatinib mesylate therapy. Blood 2003;101:3794–800.
36. O'Dwyer ME, Mauro MJ, Blasdel C, et al. Clonal evolution and lack of cytogenetic response are adverse prognostic factors for hematologic relapse of chronic phase CML patients treated with imatinib mesylate. Blood 2004;103: 451–5.
37. Willis SG, Lange T, Demehri S, et al. High-sensitivity detection of BCR-ABL kinase domain mutations in imatinib-naive patients: correlation with clonal cytogenetic evolution but not response to therapy. Blood 2005;106:2128–37.
38. Marktel S, Marin D, Foot N, et al. Chronic myeloid leukemia in chronic phase responding to imatinib: the occurrence of additional cytogenetic abnormalities predicts disease progression. Haematologica 2003;88:260–7.
39. Deininger MW. Cytogenetic studies in patients on imatinib. Semin Hematol 2003; 40:50–5.
40. Baccarani M, Cortes J, Pane F, et al. Chronic myeloid leukemia: an update of concepts and management recommendations of European LeukemiaNet. J Clin Oncol 2009;27:6041–51.

41. Verma D, Kantarjian H, Shan J, et al. Survival outcomes for clonal evolution in chronic myeloid leukemia patients on second generation tyrosine kinase inhibitor therapy. Cancer 2010;116:2673–81.

42. Yong AS, Szydlo RM, Goldman JM, et al. Molecular profiling of CD34+ cells identifies low expression of CD7, along with high expression of proteinase 3 or elastase, as predictors of longer survival in patients with CML. Blood 2006;107:205–12.

43. Radich JP, Dai H, Mao M, et al. Gene expression changes associated with progression and response in chronic myeloid leukemia. Proc Natl Acad Sci U S A 2006;103:2794–9.

44. McWeeney SK, Pemberton LC, Loriaux MM, et al. A gene expression signature of CD34+ cells to predict major cytogenetic response in chronic-phase chronic myeloid leukemia patients treated with imatinib. Blood 2010;115:315–25.

45. Zhang WW, Cortes JE, Yao H, et al. Predictors of primary imatinib resistance in chronic myelogenous leukemia are distinct from those in secondary imatinib resistance. J Clin Oncol 2009;27:3642–9.

46. Zheng C, Li L, Haak M, et al. Gene expression profiling of CD34+ cells identifies a molecular signature of chronic myeloid leukemia blast crisis. Leukemia 2006; 20:1028–34.

47. Oehler VG, Yeung KY, Choi YE, et al. The derivation of diagnostic markers of chronic myeloid leukemia progression from microarray data. Blood 2009;114:3292–8.

48. Khorashad JS, De Melo VA, Fiegler H, et al. Multiple sub-microscopic genomic lesions are a universal feature of chronic myeloid leukaemia at diagnosis. Leukemia 2008;22:1806–7.

49. Hosoya N, Sanada M, Nannya Y, et al. Genomewide screening of DNA copy number changes in chronic myelogenous leukemia with the use of high-resolution array-based comparative genomic hybridization. Genes Chromosomes Cancer 2006;45:482–94.

50. Boultwood J, Perry J, Zaman R, et al. High-density single nucleotide polymorphism array analysis and ASXL1 gene mutation screening in chronic myeloid leukemia during disease progression. Leukemia 2010;24:1139–45.

51. Joha S, Dauphin V, Lepretre F, et al. Genomic characterization of Imatinib resistance in CD34+ cell populations from chronic myeloid leukaemia patients. Leuk Res 2011;35:448–58.

52. Nadarajan VS, Phan CL, Ang CH, et al. Identification of copy number alterations by array comparative genomic hybridization in patients with late chronic or accelerated phase chronic myeloid leukemia treated with imatinib mesylate. Int J Hematol 2011;93:465–73.

53. Deluche L, Joha S, Corm S, et al. Cryptic and partial deletions of PRDM16 and RUNX1 without t(1;21)(p36;q22) and/or RUNX1-PRDM16 fusion in a case of progressive chronic myeloid leukemia: a complex chromosomal rearrangement of underestimated frequency in disease progression? Genes Chromosomes Cancer 2008;47:1110–7.

54. Nowak D, Ogawa S, Muschen M, et al. SNP array analysis of tyrosine kinase inhibitor-resistant chronic myeloid leukemia identifies heterogeneous secondary genomic alterations. Blood 2010;115:1049–53.

55. Schultheis B, Szydlo R, Mahon FX, et al. Analysis of total phosphotyrosine levels in CD34+ cells from CML patients to predict the response to imatinib mesylate treatment. Blood 2005;105:4893–4.

56. Hamilton A, Elrick L, Myssina S, et al. BCR-ABL activity and its response to drugs can be determined in CD34+ CML stem cells by CrkL phosphorylation status using flow cytometry. Leukemia 2006;20:1035–9.

57. Hamilton A, Alhashimi F, Myssina S, et al. Optimization of methods for the detection of BCR-ABL activity in Philadelphia-positive cells. Exp Hematol 2009;37: 395–401.
58. Copland M, Hamilton A, Elrick LJ, et al. Dasatinib (BMS-354825) targets an earlier progenitor population than imatinib in primary CML but does not eliminate the quiescent fraction. Blood 2006;107:4532–9.
59. Khorashad JS, Wagner S, Greener L, et al. The level of BCR-ABL1 kinase activity before treatment does not identify chronic myeloid leukemia patients who fail to achieve a complete cytogenetic response on imatinib. Haematologica 2009; 94(6):861–4.
60. White D, Saunders V, Grigg A, et al. Measurement of in vivo BCR-ABL kinase inhibition to monitor imatinib-induced target blockade and predict response in chronic myeloid leukemia. J Clin Oncol 2007;25:4445–51.
61. Cilloni D, Messa F, Gottardi E, et al. Sensitivity to imatinib therapy may be predicted by testing Wilms tumor gene expression and colony growth after a short in vitro incubation. Cancer 2004;101:979–88.
62. Jordanides NE, Jorgensen HG, Holyoake TL, et al. Functional ABCG2 is overexpressed on primary CML CD34+ cells and is inhibited by imatinib mesylate. Blood 2006;108:1370–3.
63. Engler JR, Frede A, Saunders VA, et al. Chronic myeloid leukemia CD34+ cells have reduced uptake of imatinib due to low OCT-1 activity. Leukemia 2010;24: 765–70.
64. Hatziieremia S, Jordanides NE, Holyoake TL, et al. Inhibition of MDR1 does not sensitize primitive chronic myeloid leukemia CD34+ cells to imatinib. Exp Hematol 2009;37:692–700.
65. Dohse M, Scharenberg C, Shukla S, et al. Comparison of ATP-binding cassette transporter interactions with the tyrosine kinase inhibitors imatinib, nilotinib, and dasatinib. Drug Metab Dispos 2010;38:1371–80.
66. Thomas J, Wang L, Clark RE, et al. Active transport of imatinib into and out of cells: implications for drug resistance. Blood 2004;104:3739–45.
67. Wang L, Giannoudis A, Lane S, et al. Expression of the uptake drug transporter hOCT1 is an important clinical determinant of the response to imatinib in chronic myeloid leukemia. Clin Pharmacol Ther 2008;83:258–64.
68. White DL, Saunders VA, Dang P, et al. Most CML patients who have a suboptimal response to imatinib have low OCT-1 activity: higher doses of imatinib may overcome the negative impact of low OCT-1 activity. Blood 2007;110: 4064–72.
69. White DL, Dang P, Engler J, et al. Functional activity of the OCT-1 protein is predictive of long-term outcome in patients with chronic-phase chronic myeloid leukemia treated with imatinib. J Clin Oncol 2010;28:2761–7.
70. Bazeos A, Marin D, Reid AG, et al. hOCT1 transcript levels and single nucleotide polymorphisms as predictive factors for response to imatinib in chronic myeloid leukemia. Leukemia 2010;24:1243–5.
71. Hu S, Franke RM, Filipski KK, et al. Interaction of imatinib with human organic ion carriers. Clin Cancer Res 2008;14:3141–8.
72. Marin D, Bazeos A, Mahon FX, et al. Adherence is the critical factor for achieving molecular responses in patients with chronic myeloid leukemia who achieve complete cytogenetic responses on imatinib. J Clin Oncol 2010;28: 2381–8.
73. Crossman LC, Druker BJ, Deininger MW, et al. hOCT 1 and resistance to imatinib. Blood 2005;106:1133–4.

74. Davies A, Jordanides NE, Giannoudis A, et al. Nilotinib concentration in cell lines and primary CD34(+) chronic myeloid leukemia cells is not mediated by active uptake or efflux by major drug transporters. Leukemia 2009;23:1999–2006.

75. Giannoudis A, Davies A, Lucas CM, et al. Effective dasatinib uptake may occur without human organic cation transporter 1 (hOCT1): implications for the treatment of imatinib-resistant chronic myeloid leukemia. Blood 2008;112:3348–54.

76. Fava C, Saglio G. Can we and should we improve on frontline imatinib therapy for chronic myeloid leukemia? Semin Hematol 2010;47:319–26.

77. Cortes J, Hochhaus A, Hughes T, et al. Front-line and salvage therapies with tyrosine kinase inhibitors and other treatments in chronic myeloid leukemia. J Clin Oncol 2011;29:524–31.

78. Lucas CM, Wang L, Austin GM, et al. A population study of imatinib in chronic myeloid leukaemia demonstrates lower efficacy than in clinical trials. Leukemia 2008;22:1963–6.

79. Hochhaus A, O'Brien SG, Guilhot F, et al. Six-year follow-up of patients receiving imatinib for the first line treatment of chronic myeloid leukemia. Leukemia 2009; 23:1054–61.

80. Redaelli S, Piazza R, Rostagno R, et al. Activity of bosutinib, dasatinib, and nilotinib against 18 imatinib-resistant BCR/ABL mutants. J Clin Oncol 2009;27:469–71.

81. O'Hare T, Walters DK, Stoffregen EP, et al. In vitro activity of Bcr-Abl inhibitors AMN107 and BMS-354825 against clinically relevant imatinib-resistant Abl kinase domain mutants. Cancer Res 2005;65:4500–5.

82. Azam M, Latek RR, Daley GQ. Mechanisms of autoinhibition and STI-571/imatinib resistance revealed by mutagenesis of BCR-ABL. Cell 2003;112:831–43.

83. Shah N, Nicoll J, Nagar B, et al. Multiple BCR-ABL kinase domain mutations confer polyclonal resistance to the tyrosine kinase inhibitor imatinib (STI571) in chronic phase and blast crisis chronic myeloid leukemia. Cancer Cell 2002; 2:117–223.

84. von Bubnoff N, Schneller F, Peschel C, et al. BCR-ABL gene mutations in relation to clinical resistance of Philadelphia-chromosome-positive leukaemia to STI571: a prospective study. Lancet 2002;359:487–91.

85. Gorre ME, Mohammed M, Ellwood K, et al. Clinical resistance to STI-571 cancer therapy caused by BCR-ABL gene mutation or amplification. Science 2001;293: 876–80.

86. Bradeen HA, Eide CA, O'Hare T, et al. Comparison of imatinib, dasatinib (BMS-354825), and nilotinib (AMN107) in an N-ethyl-N-nitrosourea (ENU)-based mutagenesis screen: high efficacy of drug combinations. Blood 2006;108(7):2332–8.

87. Ernst T, Erben P, Muller MC, et al. Dynamics of BCR-ABL mutated clones prior to hematologic or cytogenetic resistance to imatinib. Haematologica 2008;93:186–92.

88. Khorashad JS, Milojkovic D, Mehta P, et al. In vivo kinetics of kinase domain mutations in CML patients treated with dasatinib after failing imatinib. Blood 2008;111:2378–81.

89. Soverini S, Colarossi S, Gnani A, et al. Resistance to dasatinib in Philadelphia-positive leukemia patients and the presence or the selection of mutations at residues 315 and 317 in the BCR-ABL kinase domain. Haematologica 2007;92:401–4.

90. Pfeifer H, Wassmann B, Pavlova A, et al. Kinase domain mutations of BCR-ABL frequently precede imatinib-based therapy and give rise to relapse in patients with de novo Philadelphia-positive acute lymphoblastic leukemia (Ph+ ALL). Blood 2007;110:727–34.

91. Branford S, Rudzki Z, Walsh S, et al. Detection of BCR-ABL mutations in patients with CML treated with imatinib is virtually always accompanied by clinical

resistance, and mutations in the ATP phosphate-binding loop (P-loop) are associated with a poor prognosis. Blood 2003;102:276–83.

92. Griswold IJ, Macpartlin M, Bumm T, et al. Kinase domain mutants of Bcr-Abl exhibit altered transformation potency, kinase activity, and substrate utilization, irrespective of sensitivity to imatinib. Mol Cell Biol 2006;26:6082–93.

93. Khorashad J, de Lavallade H, Apperley J, et al. The finding of kinase domain mutations in chronic phase CML patients responding to imatinib may identify those at high risk of disease progression. J Clin Oncol 2008;26:4806–13.

94. Chu S, Xu H, Shah NP, et al. Detection of BCR-ABL kinase mutations in CD34+ cells from chronic myelogenous leukemia patients in complete cytogenetic remission on imatinib mesylate treatment. Blood 2005;105:2093–8.

95. Soverini S, Gnani A, Colarossi S, et al. Philadelphia-positive patients who already harbor imatinib-resistant Bcr-Abl kinase domain mutations have a higher likelihood of developing additional mutations associated with resistance to second- or third-line tyrosine kinase inhibitors. Blood 2009;114:2168–71.

96. Skaggs BJ, Gorre ME, Ryvkin A, et al. Phosphorylation of the ATP-binding loop directs oncogenicity of drug-resistant BCR-ABL mutants. Proc Natl Acad Sci U S A 2006;103:19466–71.

97. Branford S, Melo JV, Hughes TP. Selecting optimal second-line tyrosine kinase inhibitor therapy for chronic myeloid leukemia patients after imatinib failure—does the BCR-ABL mutation status really matter? Blood 2009;114(27):5426–35.

98. Laneuville P, Dilea C, Yin OQ, et al. Comparative In vitro cellular data alone are insufficient to predict clinical responses and guide the choice of BCR-ABL inhibitor for treating imatinib-resistant chronic myeloid leukemia. J Clin Oncol 2010; 28:e169–71.

99. Nicolini FE, Mauro MJ, Martinelli G, et al. Epidemiologic study on survival of chronic myeloid leukemia and Ph(+) acute lymphoblastic leukemia patients with BCR-ABL T315I mutation. Blood 2009;114:5271–8.

100. Azam M, Seeliger MA, Gray NS, et al. Activation of tyrosine kinases by mutation of the gatekeeper threonine. Nat Struct Mol Biol 2008;15:1109–18.

101. Hanfstein B, Muller MC, Kreil S, et al. Dynamics of mutant BCR-ABL-positive clones after cessation of tyrosine kinase inhibitor therapy. Haematologica 2011;96:360–6.

102. de Lavallade H, Khorashad JS, Davis HP, et al. Interferon-{alpha} or homoharringtonine as salvage treatment for chronic myeloid leukemia patients who acquire the T315I BCR-ABL mutation. Blood 2007;110:2779–80.

103. O'Hare T, Shakespeare WC, Zhu X, et al. AP24534, a pan-BCR-ABL inhibitor for chronic myeloid leukemia, potently inhibits the T315I mutant and overcomes mutation-based resistance. Cancer Cell 2009;16:401–12.

104. Cortes J, Talpaz M, Bixby D, et al. A phase 1 trial of oral ponatinib (AP24534) in patients with refractory chronic myelogenous leukemia (CML) and other hematologic malignancies: emerging safety and clinical response findings. ASH Annual Meeting Abstracts. Orlando (FL), December 4–7, 2010;116: p. 210.

105. Daghistani M, Marin D, Khorashad JS, et al. EVI-1 oncogene expression predicts survival in chronic-phase CML patients resistant to imatinib treated with second-generation tyrosine kinase inhibitors. Blood 2010;116: 6014–7.

106. Mahon FX, Rea D, Guilhot J, et al. Discontinuation of imatinib in patients with chronic myeloid leukaemia who have maintained complete molecular remission for at least 2 years: the prospective, multicentre Stop Imatinib (STIM) trial. Lancet Oncol 2010;11:1029–35.

Chronic Myelogenous Leukemia: Role of Stem Cell Transplant in the Imatinib Era

Nitin Jain, MD, Koen van Besien, MD*

KEYWORDS

• Chronic myelogenous leukemia • Tyrosine kinase inhibitors
• Imatinib • Allogeneic stem cell transplant

Chronic myelogenous leukemia (CML), characterized by the reciprocal translocation between chromosomes 9 and 22, t(9;22)(q34;q11), is the poster child for targeted therapies in human malignancies.[1] Tyrosine kinase inhibitors (TKIs) such as imatinib have changed the natural history of the disease and are now well established as front-line therapy for CML patients.[2] This fortunate change in treatment options has also significantly altered the role of allogeneic stem cell transplant (allo-SCT) for CML patients. Thus, the role of transplantation in CML can be divided into the pre-TKI era (before early 2000's) and the current era where the use of TKIs is virtually ubiquitous in CML patients.

ROLE OF ALLO-SCT IN CML—PRE-TKI ERA

The demonstration in the late 1970s that syngeneic (twin) donor transplant leads to the disappearance of Philadelphia chromosome established the paradigm of transplantation as curative therapy for chronic myelogenous leukemia (CML).[3] Many studies in the early 1980s established the curative potential of allo-SCT for CML,[4–6] and allo-SCT became the treatment of choice for young patients with CML and a human leukocyte antigen (HLA)-identical donor. Up to the early 1990s, chronic-phase (CP) CML was the most common indication for allo-SCT worldwide.[7] It was also the most effective treatment for patients with advanced-stage CML, though the results in accelerated phase (AP) and blast phase (BP) CML were considerably worse than those in CP because of increased rates of recurrence and of treatment-related mortality (TRM).[8,9] Practically all transplants used bone marrow (BM) as the stem cell source, and conditioning usually consisted of cyclophosphamide and total body irradiation (TBI). The initial

Section of Hematology/Oncology, Department of Medicine, University of Chicago, 5841 South Maryland Avenue, Chicago, IL 60637, USA
* Corresponding author. Weill Cornell Medical College, 520 East 70th Street, St L303, New York, NY 10021.
E-mail address: Kov9001@med.cornell.edu

Hematol Oncol Clin N Am 25 (2011) 1025–1048
doi:10.1016/j.hoc.2011.09.003
0889-8588/11/$ – see front matter © 2011 Elsevier Inc. All rights reserved.

studies used HLA-matched sibling donors (MSD); more recent ones also included unrelated donors (URD). Some of the most important studies are summarized in **Table 1**. Relapse rates were low for patients transplanted in CP, but there was a considerable incidence of treatment-related complications and treatment-related deaths. Goldman and colleagues[10] analyzed 450 patients with CP CML who received MSD allo-SCT and reported 3-year TRM, relapse rate, and overall survival (OS) ranging from 29% to 53%, 9% to 14%, and 45% to 67%, respectively, depending on the pretransplant treatment and interval from the diagnosis to the transplant. Robin and colleagues[11] reported long-term outcomes of 102 CP patients who underwent myeloablative allo-SCT from an HLA-matched sibling using TBI/cyclophosphamide or busulfan/cyclophosphamide conditioning and cyclosporine-based graft versus host disease (GVHD) prophylaxis. The 15-year relapse rate, TRM, and OS were 8%, 46%, and 53%, respectively. Hansen and colleagues[12] reported outcomes on 196 patients with CP CML who received URD allo-SCT between 1985 and 1994 with the use of cyclophosphamide/TBI myeloablative conditioning. At 5 years the relapse rate was 10%, nonrelapse mortality (NRM) 44%, and OS 57%. Acute grade II to IV GVHD occurred in 77% patients and chronic extensive GVHD in 67% patients.

While most of the deaths after the allo-SCT occur within the first 5 years, some patients also succumb to late sequelae. Goldman and colleagues,[13] analyzing Center for International Blood and Marrow Transplant Research (CIBMTR) data, reported outcomes on 2444 patients who received myeloablative allo-SCT in CP1 and survived in continuous complete remission for 5 years or longer. The OS for the entire patient population was 94% at 10 years and 87% at 15 years. Compared with the age-, sex-, and race-matched general population, patients who had survived 5 years after allo-SCT still had a 2.5-times higher risk of death at 10 years, due to long-term complications of the allo-SCT. The most common causes of late deaths were organ failure (17%), infection (15%), GVHD (14%), disease relapse (7%), and secondary malignancies (7%). The mortality rates, however, for those surviving at 15-years after allo-SCT approached that of the general population. The cumulative incidence of relapse for the entire cohort was 4% at 10 years and 7% at 15 years after allo-SCT.

In the pre–tyrosine kinase inhibitor (TKI) era, there was a debate on appropriate age limits and timing of allo-SCT versus noncurative treatments with moderate efficacy, such as interferon (IFN) or IFN-cytarabine combination. The toxicity of myeloablative transplants was such that they were restricted to patients without significant comorbidities and mostly to those younger than 60 years. As the median age of diagnosis of CML is 65 years in the United States,[14] the majority of patients were not eligible for the myeloablative transplant.

Many different approaches were tested to circumvent this limitation, including T-cell–depleted transplants, autologous transplants, and reduced-intensity conditioning (RIC). Experience with syngeneic transplants had shown that high-dose conditioning followed by the infusion of a tumor-free graft can induce durable remission. Based on this concept, several groups in the late 1980s explored the use of in vitro T-cell depletion to avoid both acute and chronic GVHD.[15,16] These types of transplant were safer and were effective in preventing GVHD. Unfortunately they were also associated with high rates of graft failure, opportunistic infections, and increased rates of disease relapse, due to lack of induction of the graft versus leukemia (GvL) effect. In one such series, reporting on the outcomes of 405 patients in CP CML reported to the CIBMTR, patients with T-cell–depleted allo-SCT had 3-year probability of relapse of 48% compared with 9% with non–T-cell–depleted allo-SCT.[15]

An alternative approach used autologous transplants rather than allo-SCT. Several studies evaluated induction of remission with chemotherapy followed by stem cell

Table 1
Myeloablative conditioning allogeneic stem cell transplant in chronic myelogenous leukemia

Authors	No. of Patients	Disease Phase	Donor Source	Conditioning Regimen	TRM	Relapse Rate	GVHD	OS
Thomas et al[8]	167	CP1 67, CP2 12, AP 46, BP 42	MSD	TBI/CY	43% for CP1	18% for CP1	51% chronic GVHD among long-term survivors	At 3 y: CP 58%, AP 14%
Goldman et al[10]	450	CP	MSD	TBI/CY or Bu/CY	29%–53%	9%–14%		45%–67% at 3 y
Hansen et al[12]	196	CP	URD	TBI/CY	43%	10% at 5 y	Acute grade II–IV GVHD: 77%, extensive chronic GVHD: 67%	57% at 5 y
Radich et al[97]	131	CP	HLA-matched relative	Targeted Bu/CY	14%	8% at 3 y	Acute grade II–IV GVHD: 65%, extensive chronic GVHD: 60%	86% at 3 y
Robin et al[11]	102	CP	MSD	TBI/CY or Bu/CY	46% at 15 y	8% at 15 y	Chronic extensive GVHD 49%	53% at 15 y

Abbreviations: AP, accelerated phase; BP, blast phase; Bu, busulfan; CP, chronic phase; CY, cyclophosphamide; GVHD, graft versus host disease; MSD, HLA-matched sibling donor; OS, overall survival; TBI, total body irradiation; TRM, transplant-related mortality; URD, unrelated donors.

harvest in cytogenetic remission and autologous transplantation.[17–21] These studies, which used unmanipulated grafts or a variety of ex vivo or in vivo purging methods to decrease the contamination by malignant clone, are now merely of historical interest, but they did show that duration of remissions correlates with the extent of residual stem cell contamination, which implies that autologous transplant with tumor-free grafts might be a curative procedure.[22] McGlave and colleagues[20] reported pooled data on 200 CML patients who underwent autologous transplant, with most patients receiving unmanipulated grafts. Median survival for the entire group was 42 months (CP: not reached; AP: 35.9 months; BP: 4.1 months). Most surviving patients, however, had evidence of persistent disease by cytogenetic or hematological parameters.

Kolb and colleagues[23] were the first to show that donor lymphocyte infusion (DLI) could reliably induce remission in those relapsing with CML after allo-SCT, an observation that has been extensively reproduced.[24–27] This finding, along with the observation that GvL effect plays an important role in disease control after allo-SCT[28–32] and concerns over the potential toxicities of conventional myeloablation, led many groups in the last decade to use lower doses of the conditioning regimens (so-called RIC or nonmyeloablative conditioning) with the aim of decreasing NRM and using the GvL effect to maintain the disease control (**Table 2**).[9,28–31,33–44] Most of these studies were initiated in the pre-TKI era. After the introduction of imatinib, many of these studies had difficulty accruing patients, and few observations have been confirmed in large clinical trials.

STEM CELL TRANSPLANT IN THE ERA OF TYROSINE KINASE INHIBITORS
The Changing Paradigm

Given its superior efficacy, ease of administration, and the lack of significant side effects, imatinib was rapidly adopted as the first-line medical therapy in CP CML patients. However, clinicians across the globe also rapidly adopted the oral TKI therapy as a preferred alternative to transplant. Imatinib was approved by the United States Food and Drug Administration (FDA) in October 2001. The decline in the number of allo-SCT for CML started before FDA approval, and certainly before the availability of long-term follow-up data. Gratwohl and colleagues[45] reported on behalf of the European Group for Blood and Marrow Transplantation (EBMT) outcomes of all CML patients reported to the EBMT between 1980 and 2004. The number of allo-SCT in Europe peaked in 1999 with 1396 transplants, with a subsequent decrease to 791 allo-SCT in 2003 and 434 allo-SCT in 2007, a 69% decrease.[45,46] These investigators also reported a significant increase in the proportion of URD transplants (7% in 1980–1990 to 36% in 2000–2003), increasing use of peripheral blood (PB) as a source of stem cells (21% in 1990-2000 vs 53% in 2000-2003) and the use of RIC regimens.[45,46] Bacher and colleagues[47] reported 72% decrease in number of CML transplants from 1998 to 2004 in Germany, with a larger percentage decrease in patients undergoing allo-SCT in CP1. A similar pattern was reported by CIBMTR whereby the reported number of allo-SCT decreased from 617 in 1998 to 223 in 2003.[48] The majority of the decrease in the transplant numbers is for CP1 patients, for whom TKIs have become the front-line standard treatment. The number of patients transplanted in AP/BP has remained relatively stable.[48]

Economic factors may also have an impact on the choice between allo-SCT and TKI therapy, especially in the developing countries. Ruiz-Argüelles and colleagues[49] reported data on 24 patients transplanted in CP1 using MSD and RIC in 4 Latin American countries; they mentioned the cost of allo-SCT in Mexico would be equal to approximately 200 days of imatinib 400 mg daily, thus making the case for allo-SCT.[49] Similar observations were made by Gratwohl and colleagues[50] when they analyzed the EBMT survey data; they noticed that the rates of allo-SCT fell after the introduction of imatinib in high-income countries in Europe but remained relatively stable for the lower-income countries, indicating persistent reliance on the "one-time" cost of allo-SCT as compared with expensive potentially "life-long" TKI therapy.[50]

ALLO-SCT COMPARED WITH IMATINIB AS FRONT-LINE THERAPY IN CHRONIC PHASE

As imatinib was rapidly adopted as a standard front-line therapy for CP CML, with excellent results, randomized clinical trials to prove the superiority of imatinib to allo-SCT were considered unjustifiable. As a result, only indirect evidence exists with which to compare the two modalities. In a study by the German CML group, newly diagnosed CP CML patients with a matched siblings were offered matched-related donor allo-SCT; all others were given the best available drug therapy (IFN plus hydroxyurea at the time of initiation of this study).[51] This type of treatment assignment based on donor availability is sometimes called genetic randomization. With a median observation time of 8.9 years, the survival was superior for patients in the drug treatment arm ($P = .049$), particularly in the low-risk patients. The survival difference was most pronounced at 3 years with the two curves merging only at approximately 8 years, given steady disease progression in the drug treatment arm. Of note, two-thirds of the patients in the drug therapy arm were over time switched to imatinib because of failure of or intolerance to IFN/hydroxyurea. These data, though debated at the time, were the first to indicate superiority of drug treatment over allo-SCT in CP CML patients and to provide a compelling argument for superiority of TKI therapy as front-line treatment for CP CML patients in comparison with allo-SCT. In another retrospective analysis reported by Bittencourt and colleagues,[52] CP1 CML patients who failed or were intolerant to IFN received either imatinib as second-line therapy (n = 174) or allo-SCT (n = 90) based on availability of donor and Sokal score. The imatinib group had significantly improved event-free survival (EFS) and OS at 5 years compared with the allo-SCT group, again indicating superiority of the imatinib in this setting.

A third more recent study from the German CML Study IV group took a slightly different approach. This group reported interim outcomes on 1242 CML patients who underwent 5-arm treatment randomization (imatinib 400 mg daily vs imatinib plus IFN vs imatinib plus cytarabine vs imatinib post-IFN failure vs imatinib 800 mg daily).[53] Based on predefined transplantation criteria (high Hasford score and/or low EBMT score, imatinib-failure or AP/BP), 84 of these 1242 patients underwent allo-SCT between 2003 and 2008 (23% in CP1 as an elective option, 44% after imatinib failure in CP1, and 33% in AP/BP). The median age at the time of transplantation was 37 years (range, 16–62 years). All except 3 patients received imatinib pretransplantation. Seventy percent of CP patients and 42% of AP/BP patients had achieved cytogenetic remission at the time of transplantation. Three-year OS was 91% for patients in CP and 59% for patients in AP/BP. In the matched-pair analysis, survival at 3 years was similar for the patients who underwent allo-SCT in CP1 versus those who were treated with imatinib alone, though those assigned to transplant had a higher risk score. The investigators draw attention to the very low TRM of 8% in this study, which they attribute to improvements in supportive care, and also speculate that imatinib-induced reduction of tumor burden prior to transplant may have favorably influenced outcomes.

Although the debate over front-line therapy for adults with CP CML has been settled in favor of TKI therapy, whether the same could be said for pediatric patients with CML is not entirely clear. Cwynarski and colleagues[54] reported retrospective EBMT data on

Table 2
Reduced-intensity conditioning allogeneic stem cell transplant in chronic myelogenous leukemia

Authors	No. of Patients	Median Age	Time Period	Disease Phase	Donor Type	Donor Source	Median Follow-Up (mo)	Conditioning Regimen	Use of Prior Imatinib	TRM	Relapse Rate	GVHD	OS
Or et al[35]	24	35	1996–2001	CP1	MSD (n = 18), father (n = 1), URD (n = 5)	PB	37	Flu/Bu (n = 19), Flu/Bu/ATG (n = 5)	No	0% at 100 d, 4% at 1 y	0%	Acute (grade II–IV) 71%, Chronic 54%	85%
Das et al[34]	17	34	1998–2000	CP1 (n = 16), AP (n = 1)	MSD	BM (n = 3), PB (n = 14)	30	Flu/Bu/ATG (n = 11), Flu/Bu/TBI (n = 6)	No	12% at 100 d	—	Acute (grade II–IV) 41%, Chronic 65%	47% (1 y)
Bornhauser et al[144]	44	52	NR	CP (n = 26), AP (n = 11), BP (n = 7)	MSD (n = 19), URD (n = 15)	BM (n = 15), PB (n = 29)	—	Flu/Bu (ATG in 34 patients)	No	NR	NR	Acute (grade II–IV) 43%, Chronic not reported	14.8 mo
Weisser et al[36]	35 (included patients only ≥45 y)	51	—	CP1 (n = 26), CP2/AP (n = 9)	MSD (n = 19), URD (n = 16)	BM (n = 31), PB (n = 4)	30	TBI 8 Gy/Flu/CY/ATG	No	11% at 100 d, 28.5% at 1 y	8% CP1, 33% for CP2/AP	Acute (grade II–IV) 48%, Chronic extensive 23%	69% at 2 y
Crawley et al[9]	186	50	1994–2002	CP1 (63%), CP2 (14%), AP/BP (23%)	MSD (60%), URD (25%)	BM (28.5%), PB (71.5%)	35	Variety of regimens; Flu/Bu/ATG in 40%	8%	3.8% (100 d); 13.3% (1 y); 18.9% (2 y)	47% at 3 y	Acute (grade II–IV) 30%, Chronic 42%	54% at 3 y
Kerbauy et al[37]	24	57.5	1998–2003	CP (n = 14), CP2 (n = 4), AP (n = 6)	Matched related donors	PB	36	TBI 2 Gy alone (n = 8); TBI/Flu (n = 16)	Yes (n = 7)	4% at 100 d	For CP1: 22% at 2 y	Acute (grade II–IV) 46%, Chronic 57%	For CP1: 70% at 2 y

Study													
Kebriaei et al[38]	64	52	1996–2005	CP1 20%, CP2 27%, AP/BP 53%	Matched related 47%, URD 47%	BM 59%, PB 41%	84	All regimens Flu-based; Flu/Mel 47%	14%	TRM at 100 d 33%, at 1 y 38%	34%	Acute (grade II–IV) 31%, Chronic 31%	For CP, OS at 2 and 5 y was 66% and 48%
Luo et al[41]	28	26	2005–2007	CP1	HLA-identical donors	BM (n = 7); PB (n = 21)	23	Flu/Bu/ATG; prophylactic imatinib from day 100 until 1 y	Yes, all patients	3.6% at 100 d, 14.3% at 1 y	32%	Acute (grade II–IV) 8% (no grade II–IV), Chronic 48%	81% at 3 y
Olavarria et al[198]	22	49	NR	CP1	HLA-identical sibling	PB stem cells	36	Flu/Bu alemtuzumab Patients received posttransplant imatinib	Yes (50% patients)	0% at 100 d, 4% at 1 y	68% (all after posttransplant imatinib discontinuation)	Acute (grade II–IV) 5%, Chronic none	87% at 3 y
Champlin et al[39]	33	41	—	CP1 (n = 16), CP2/AP (n = 17)	—	—	29	Flu/Bu/ATG Patients with residual disease received planned imatinib and DLI	Yes, all patients	0% at 100 d	41% for AP/BP, none in CP	Acute (grade II–IV) 21%	76%
Poire et al[42]	9	61	2002–2007	CP1 (n = 3), CP2 (n = 2), AP (n = 1), BP (n = 3)	MSD (n = 7), URD 8/8 match (n = 1), URD 7/8 match (n = 1)	PB	—	Flu/Bu alemtuzumab (n = 4), Flu/Mel/alemtuzumab (n = 4), Bu/CY/alemtuzumab (n = 1)	Yes, all patients (4 patients prior dasatinib also)	0% at 100 d, 33% at 1 y	—	Grade II–IV acute GVHD (45%) (none grade III–IV)	—

Abbreviations: AP, accelerated phase; ATG, antithymocyte globulin; BM, bone marrow; BP, blast phase; Bu, busulfan; CP, chronic phase; CY, cyclophosphamide; DLI, donor lymphocyte infusion; Flu, fludarabine; Flu, fludarabine; GVHD, graft versus host disease; Mel, melphalan; MSD, HLA-matched sibling donor; OS, overall survival; PB, peripheral blood; TBI, total body irradiation; TRM, transplant-related mortality; URD, unrelated donor.

the outcomes of 314 children (median age 14 years) who underwent allo-SCT for CML in the pre-imatinib era (between 1985 and 2001). The donor was an HLA-matched sibling in 58%, and 81% were in CP1 at the time of allo-SCT. The source of stem cells was BM for all patients. For CP1 patients, 3-year OS, TRM, and relapse rate for those receiving sibling donor versus URD was 75%, 20%, 17%, and 65%, 31%, 13%, respectively. Grade II to IV acute GVHD occurred significantly more in the URD group (52% vs 37% for sibling donors). Suttorp and colleagues[55] reported 10-year prospective follow-up data on 176 children who underwent allo-SCT for CML from year 1995 to 2004 (median age 12.4 years). At the time of allo-SCT, 82% were in CP1 and 66% underwent matched sibling allo-SCT. For CP1 patients, OS was 64% with significantly better OS in the matched sibling group (OS 87% compared with 52% in matched URD transplant group, $P = .002$). Thus the outcomes in pediatric patients appear superior to those in the adults. Data with use of imatinib in children is limited and again, as is true for adults, very long-term data on imatinib use is unavailable. However, as is the case with adults, the current consensus is to use imatinib as front-line therapy for CML in children.[56]

At present, 3 broad groups of patients are considered to benefit from allo-SCT:

1. Those in AP or BP
2. Those failing/intolerant to TKI therapy
3. Those with TKI-resistant mutations such as T315I mutation.

Patients in AP/BP

Long-term outcomes of patients treated with single-agent imatinib for advanced-phase disease range from an OS of 37 to 47 months for AP, and of approximately 7 months for BP.[57–59] Second-generation TKIs are superior to imatinib, but are not considered curative in advanced-phase CML. Allo-SCT provides the only potential for long-term survival for these individuals. However, the outcomes after allo-SCT for this group of patients remain suboptimal, especially for BP disease. Gratwohl and colleagues[45] reported 2-year OS, TRM, and relapse rate for AP and BP disease as 47%, 37%, 28%, and 16%, 50%, 38%, respectively. Jiang and colleagues[60] reported on the outcomes of AP patients who were assigned to treatment with imatinib versus an upfront allo-SCT.[60] The treatment assignment was non-randomized and based on patient's preference. The allo-SCT group had superior outcomes (6-year EFS and OS rates of 71.8% and 83.3%, respectively compared to 39.2% and 51.4%, respectively for the imatinib group). A multivariate analysis revealed that a CML duration greater than or equal to 12 months, hemoglobin less than 100 g/L, and peripheral blood blasts greater than or equal to 5% were independent poor prognostic factors for both OS and progression-free survival (PFS). When stratified by these 3 risk factors, the superiority of allo-SCT was seen in only intermediate (presence of one factor) and high-risk (presence of ≥ 2 factors) groups. Patients without any risk factor (low-risk) did equally well with imatinib or allo-SCT. Patients with advanced-phase CML remain a challenging group of patients with poor outcomes with currently available therapies, and every effort should be made to induce a second CP before allo-SCT.

Patients Who Fail TKI Therapy

As TKIs have become standard therapy for newly diagnosed CML patients, almost all patients with CML will have received imatinib and/or second-generation TKIs before proceeding with an allo-SCT. Even for patients with advanced disease, as the plans for allo-SCT are being formulated patients will usually be initiated on a TKI. Patients who have failed TKI represent the majority of those undergoing transplantation. So an important question is whether prior use of TKIs affects the transplant outcomes.

Effect of prior imatinib or second-generation TKIs on transplant outcomes

Deininger and colleagues[61] reported retrospective data on 70 patients with CML who underwent allo-SCT after imatinib treatment, and compared the outcomes with a historical control group from EBMT registry. Eighty- four percent of the patients were in AP/BP prior to imatinib, and this was reduced to 44% prior to allo-SCT. Median duration of imatinib therapy was 97 days, and the median interval from diagnosis to transplantation was 22.6 months. When compared with the historical controls, the investigators found no influence of prior imatinib use on OS, PFS, and NRM. Another study from CIBMTR evaluated 409 patients (185 patients CP1; the rest advanced disease) who received imatinib before allo-SCT in comparison with 900 patients who did not receive imatinib before allo-SCT.[62] In the multivariate model, exposure to imatinib prior to allo-SCT was associated with better OS. Leukemia-free survival (LFS) and rates of acute and chronic GVHD were similar in the two groups. For the patients beyond CP1 there was no difference in the OS, LFS, TRM, or relapse rate. Other groups have also reported that pretransplant use of imatinib is safe and is not associated with increased TRM.[63–65]

In addition, response to imatinib prior to allo-SCT has been shown to improve clinical outcomes for CP patients. Oehler and colleagues[65] reported allo-SCT outcomes of 69 patients who had received imatinib before allo-SCT. Those who had achieved major cytogenetic remission (MCyR) prior to allo-SCT had better outcome than those who did not (or who lost their cytogenetic response). The latter group had a statistically significantly higher hazard of mortality (hazard ratio 5.31, $P = .03$).

In the initial few years of the TKI era, allo-SCT was recommended after imatinib failure/intolerance.[66] At present, second-generation TKIs (dasatinib and nilotinib) have shown excellent results in imatinib failure/intolerant patients with MCyR in up to 40% to 45% patients, and as such have been approved by the FDA for this indication.[67,68] In addition, both dasatinib and nilotinib have shown excellent results as front-line therapy for CP CML, and have been recently approved by the FDA for front-line therapy.[69,70] It is therefore not surprising that most patients now will have received a second-generation TKI at the time of consideration for an allo-SCT. Second-generation TKIs have also been reported to be safe when used prior to allo-SCT.[71,72] In accordance with the aforementioned data, the recent European LeukemiaNet guidelines advocate allo-SCT after failure of a second-generation TKI (and not after only imatinib failure).[73]

Patients with TKI-Resistant Mutations

Although many mutations have been identified in the Abl kinase domain, contributing to the resistance to TKIs, threonine-to-isoleucine substitution at position 315 of Bcr-Abl fusion protein (T315I mutation) leads to resistance to all first-generation and second-generation TKIs. Given the lack of effectiveness of the TKIs, early allo-SCT is recommended for such patients.[73] Velev and colleagues[74] reported outcomes of 8 patients with T315I mutation who underwent allo-SCT. At the time of allo-SCT 2 patients were in CP1, 3 patients were in AP, and 3 patients were in CP2. The best responses after allo-SCT were complete molecular remission (CMR) in 3 patients, complete cytogenetic response (CCyR) in 4 patients, and complete hematologic response (CHR) in 1 patient. The 2 patients in CP1 at the time of allo-SCT had the best outcomes.[74] There have been other anecdotal reports of patients undergoing allo-SCT for T315I mutation, with good outcomes.[75,76] Jabbour and colleagues[77] reported allo-SCT outcomes of 19 patients who underwent allo-SCT due imatinib failure secondary to a BCR-ABL kinase domain mutation. The 2-year EFS and OS were 36% and 44%, respectively. They also reported that these outcomes were inferior (though encouraging) compared to outcomes of 28 other patients treated at the same institution with an allo-SCT for a non-mutation related imatinib failure. Nicolini and colleagues[78] reported on 64 patients with T315I mutation who underwent allo-SCT. At the time of allo-SCT, 51% of patients were in CP and 26% were in blast crisis. The 2-yr OS rate for CP, AP, and BP disease were 59%, 67% and 30%, respectively. These results are better than that achieved by non-transplant strategies,[79] though emerging data on the efficacy of third-generation TKIs such as ponatinib in T315I mutated patients may alter this argument in near future.[80]

METHODS OF TRANSPLANTATION AND PATIENT SELECTION
Prognostic Scoring Systems

Patients and physicians deciding on transplantation face an uncertain outcome, and various attempts have been made to better quantify risks and survival after allogeneic transplant. The prognostic risk scoring system developed by the EBMT is the most commonly used scoring system for patient undergoing allo-SCT for CML, and its predictive value has been validated in two independent data sets. It is based on the sum of 5 variables: donor type (0 for HLA-identical sibling donor, 1 for a matched unrelated donor); disease stage (0 for CP1, 1 for AP, and 2 for BP or higher CP); age of recipient (0 for <20 years, 1 for 20–40 years, and 2 for >40 years); sex combination (0 for all, except 1 for male recipient/female donor); and time from diagnosis to transplantation (0 for <12 months, 1 for >12 months).[81] A higher score is associated with worse TRM, OS, and relapse rate. Survival at 5 years ranges from 76% for those with EBMT score 0 to 19% for those with EBMT score 6.[81,82] Recently Pavlu and colleagues[83] used a combination of comorbidity index (HCT-CI) together with levels of C-reactive protein (CRP) to predict not just overall survival but also TRM at 100 days after transplant.[84] In the multivariate analysis both HCT-CI score greater than 0 and CRP levels greater than 9 mg/L were independent predictors for inferior OS and increased day-100 NRM. The investigators suggested that patients with HCT-CI score of zero and with normal CRP level might be candidates for early allo-SCT after imatinib failure.[83]

Source of Stem Cells: PB Versus BM

Over the past decade mobilized PB stem cells have gradually replaced BM as the preferred graft source, particularly for sibling transplants. Ease and convenience of donor collection play an important role in this shift, as do important physiologic differences between mobilized PB and BM. PB allo-SCT is associated with more rapid platelet and neutrophil engraftment and a lower risk of disease relapse, but has higher risk of acute and particularly chronic GVHD.[85–87] This finding has major implications for the outcome of allo-SCT in CML. Elmaagacli and colleagues[85] reported on the outcomes of CP1 CML patients who underwent HLA-matched sibling or partial HLA-matched family donor, and compared the outcomes of BM (n = 62) versus PB (n = 29) donor source. The investigators reported a higher rate of molecular and cytogenetic relapse with BM as a stem cell source, but did not compare OS rates. In a meta-analysis for HLA-MSD transplants, the use of PB was associated with lower relapse risk (odds ratio = 0.34, 95% confidence interval 0.2–0.58) and higher acute and chronic GVHD.[86] OS was improved with the use of PB as stem cell source in advanced-phase CML (CP2, AP, BP) compared with BM, but OS was similar for

CP1 CML patients.[86] Schmitz and colleagues[88,89] also reported long-term outcomes for PB versus BM for HLA-matched sibling transplants for the CIBMTR/EBMT data set. Contrary to the meta-analysis results reported above, relapse risk was similar for PB versus BM group and significantly higher TRM, and worse disease-free survival (DFS) and OS was seen in the CP1 group who received PB as stem cell source.[89] OS was improved for advanced-phase CML with the use of PB as stem cell source, similar to that of the meta-analysis results.

Oehler and colleagues[90] analyzed 72 CML patients who were randomized to undergo HLA-matched allo-SCT with either BM or PB as the source of donor cells. There was no statistically significant difference in the OS, incidence of acute/chronic GVHD, or NRM between the two groups.

Although the data from various reports are not entirely consistent, it is reasonable to conclude that there is little advantage to the use of unmanipulated PB stem cells in CML CP1 and that there is an increased risk for chronic GVHD. The more rapid blood count recovery and more profound GvL effects after PB stem cell transplant may, however, constitute an advantage in CML AP or BP.

Type of Donor: Sibling Versus Unrelated

Only about 25% of patients have HLA-identical siblings, and unrelated donor transplantation is a necessary alternative. In an early report from the National Marrow Donor Program reporting on AP/BP CML patients, 5-year OS for MSD was 31%, significantly better than 20% for URD ($P = .002$).[91] As typing technology and supportive care for transplant improved, so did outcomes of unrelated donor transplantation. In a 1998 study, the Seattle group reported a 74% 5-year survival for patients younger than 50 years with CP1 undergoing URD.[12] A recent report from the CIBMTR compared the outcomes of URD transplants (n = 1052) with those after MSD transplants (n = 3514) in patients receiving BM transplants for CML in CP1.[92] OS at 5 years was approximately 8% better after MSD (63%) versus 8/8 matched URD (55%). Survival was progressively worse, with greater degrees of HLA mismatch in the URD group. Thus, an MSD remains the preferred donor type, though the results for URD in early-phase CML are currently quite similar to those of MSD. For those lacking either MSD or URD, many centers currently recommend umbilical cord stem cell transplantation (UCB). Sanz and colleagues[93] recently reported the outcome of 26 patients with CML who underwent UCB SCT. At the time of transplantation 7 patients were in CP1, 11 were in CP2, 2 were in AP, and 6 were in BP. TRM was 41% for patients undergoing UCB SCT in CP1 or CP2 and 100% for patients in AP or BP. A Japanese registry study reported outcomes in 86 patients with CML who underwent UCB SCT.[94] Two-year survival for patients in CP, AP and BP was 71, 59 and 32%, respectively.

CONDITIONING REGIMEN

Classic myeloablative transplantation combining TBI with high-dose cyclophosphamide was long considered the standard conditioning regimen for allo-SCT in CML. The high-dose busulfan/cyclophosphamide regimen was developed as an alternative conditioning regimen, and in randomized studies was found to result in equivalent long-term outcomes, though the toxicity profile was slightly different.[95] Subsequently, attempts were made to "target" the busulfan dose to achieve optimal results.[96,97] More recently, the majority of groups have focused on nonmyeloablative or RIC regimens. Low-dose TBI (200 cGy) alone as a conditioning regimen was associated with an increased graft rejection in CML patients, prompting the combination with fludarabine. In the study by the Seattle group, the 2-year survival estimates for patients in CP1 (n = 14) and beyond CP1 (n = 10) were 70% and 56%, respectively.[37] Kebriaei and colleagues,[38] for the MD Anderson group, reported long-term outcomes of 64 patients, most of whom received a reduced-intensity fludarabine/melphalan combination. Thirteen patients were in CP1, 17 were in CP2, 29 were in AP, and 5 were in BP. With median follow-up of 7 years, OS and PFS were 33% and 20%, respectively, at 5 years. Incidence of TRM was 33% at 100 days and 48% at 5 years after hemopoietic SCT. In multivariate analysis, only disease stage at time of allo-SCT was significantly predictive for both OS and PFS. For CP1/2 patients PFS and TRM were 31% and 42% at 5 years, respectively. These data confirm the curative potential of RIC conditioning in CML, but the investigators also acknowledge considerable failure rates and TRM. To avoid some of the complications associated with fludarabine/melphalan-based conditioning, the authors and others have combined it with in vivo T-cell depletion using alemtuzumab. The main concern with this approach is increased risk of disease relapse, which could be countered by use of prophylactic imatinib and/or DLI posttransplant, which is discussed below.[98–100]

Treosulfan, a busulfan analogue, may have a more favorable toxicity profile, and a fludarabine/treosulfan combination has extensively been tested in Europe. Holowiecki and colleagues[101] reported on 40 patients with CML CP who underwent allo-SCT. The 2-year probability of OS, LFS, and TRM was 85%, 82%, and 15%, respectively. The cumulative incidence of hematologic relapse was only 2.5%, but 15 patients received further therapy for declining chimerism and cytogenetic recurrence. The combined cumulative incidence of hematologic and cytogenetic recurrence reached 46%. This regimen, though well tolerated, may therefore not be sufficiently antileukemic by itself to provide durable remissions, and warrants posttransplant therapy in many cases.

MONITORING AFTER ALLO-SCT

Relapse after allo-SCT remains an important clinical problem, and though most cases occur within the first few years after the allo-SCT, relapses 10 to 15 years after allo-SCT have been reported.[13] Detection of PB/BM Bcr-Abl transcript level has been shown by many groups to be predictive for disease relapse.[102–106] Kaeda and colleagues[105] reported on 243 CML patients who underwent conventional myeloablative allo-SCT and had serial monitoring by Bcr-Abl real-time polymerase chain reaction (RT-PCR) of the peripheral blood. Patients were characterized as "persistently negative" (n = 36, single low-level positive result), "fluctuating positive, low level" (n = 51, >1 positive result but never >2 consecutive positive results), "persistently positive, low level" (n = 27, persistent low levels but never >3 consecutive positive results), or "relapsed" (n = 129). The risk of relapse significantly correlated with the risk category (persistent negative: 2.7%; fluctuating positive: 20.8%; persistent positive: 30.0%), with most relapses occurring within the first 5 years after transplant.[105] The same group had previously reported the importance of quantitative RT-PCR done early (3–5 months) after allo-SCT.[106] Three-year relapse rates were reported as 16.7%, 42.9%, and 86.4% for those with negative, low-positive, and high-positive transcript levels, respectively. Therefore, serial Bcr-Abl RT-PCR monitoring is considered by many a standard clinical practice after allo-SCT, and can be used to guide therapeutic interventions. The detection of low levels of Bcr-Abl early after transplant is expected, and treatment decisions should be based on serial measurements of high or increasing levels of Bcr-Abl.[105] International efforts are ongoing to implement standardization of RT-PCR levels.[107]

PREVENTION OR EARLY TREATMENT OF DISEASE RECURRENCE WITH TKIs OR CELLULAR THERAPY POST TRANSPLANT

DLI routinely induces remissions in patients with disease recurrence after allo-SCT, and was long considered the standard treatment for patients with early disease recurrence. However, DLI carries a risk of myelosuppression and GVHD, which in turn is associated with DLI related mortality. The risk for GVHD can be modulated (but not abolished) by decreasing the dose of T cells contained in the DLI and by delaying DLI as much as possible.[26,108–110] Because of its associated risks, DLI is rarely given prophylactically but rather for treatment of molecular relapse as defined by an increasing level of Bcr-Abl. The routine induction of remission by DLI has given rise to the concept of "current leukemia-free survival," defined as the probability that a patient is alive and in remission at a given time after transplantation.[111]

Given the effectiveness of imatinib in the front-line setting and its attractive safety profile, many groups have explored the use of imatinib as a prophylactic measure after allo-SCT to prevent relapse. Carpenter and colleagues[112] treated 22 patients (7 CML patients beyond CP1 and 15 Ph+ ALL patients) with imatinib post allo-SCT at the standard dose of 400 mg daily. Imatinib was started at a median of 29 days post allo-SCT and continued for 1 year. Imatinib was safe without significant cytopenias, and did not affect the calcineurin inhibitor levels.[112] The results were encouraging, with 17 of the 22 patients in CMR after 1.3 years follow-up. Olavarria and colleagues[98] evaluated the role of imatinib after allo-SCT in 22 patients with an alemtuzumab-based RIC regimen in CP1 with HLA-MSD. Imatinib was given from day 35 to 1 year after allo-SCT, and was well tolerated. All patients achieved major molecular remission (MMR) with imatinib administration, and none had a cytogenetic relapse during the duration of imatinib use. After the planned imatinib discontinuation at 1 year, 75% of patients relapsed and all of these patients underwent DLI. With DLI, the majority regained a molecular response. Whether or not all patients should be offered imatinib as a maintenance therapy post transplant and for what duration or with which remission goal (such as MMR or CMR) remains unclear at this point. In the study by Olavarria and colleagues[98] the majority of the patients relapsed after imatinib discontinuation, indicating that imatinib may have to be continued for longer durations and that perhaps life-long treatment may be needed. It is likely that increasingly patients will be referred who have failed all available TKIs. Occasional observation of restoration of sensitivity to TKI after transplant justifies their reintroduction in that setting.[42] Still, whenever possible a TKI should be chosen with documented activity, and mutation analysis of Bcr-Abl is essential in all cases. While posttransplant imatinib seems safe, this may not be the case for all TKIs. Dasatinib in particular can cause life-threatening fluid retention and may also be quite immunosuppressive.[113]

One could also consider a synergistic combination of DLI with TKI, as suggested by Savani and colleagues.[114] Given the rapid development of novel TKIs and other drugs, it is likely that in the near future the patients referred to allo-SCT will be those who have exhausted a plethora of medical strategies. Posttransplant management is likely to change, but it is safe to predict that posttransplant cellular therapy will assume a larger role again, with their use guided by serial Bcr-Abl RT-PCR monitoring with its dosing optimized to avoid GVHD.[108]

MANAGEMENT OF HEMATOLOGIC RELAPSE AFTER ALLO-SCT

In the pre-imatinib era, DLI was the cornerstone of treatment for patients who relapse after allo-SCT.[23,27] Other therapies used commonly at that time included IFN and a second allo-SCT. With the clinical efficacy of the TKIs in the pretransplant setting, there was an increasing interest in using TKIs at the time of disease relapse after the transplant. Kantarjian and colleagues[115] reported on 28 such patients who relapsed at a median of 9 months after transplant. Of these, 13 patients had already received DLI as salvage. Overall, imatinib led to CHR in 74% and CCyR in 35% of patients, with better responses seen in CP patients. The majority of patients who had received DLI as salvage responded to imatinib. Olavarria and colleagues[116] used imatinib in 128 patients with CML relapsed after allo-SCT. Fifty of the patients had failed prior DLI. The overall CHR was 84%. The CCyR ranged from 58% for patients in CP to 22% for patients in BP. Imatinib was well tolerated, with 10% patients with worsening of underlying GVHD and no episodes of new-onset GVHD after the initiation of imatinib.[116] Hess and colleagues[117] reported outcomes of a prospective phase 2 trial in which patients in CP1 undergoing allo-SCT were treated with imatinib at the time of disease relapse (n = 37; molecular relapse n = 18, cytogenetic relapse n = 19). Imatinib was well tolerated, with only 1 patient (2.3%) with grade 1 to 2 reactivation of GVHD. Within the first 9 months, CMR was achieved in 62.2% patients (77.8% in those with molecular relapse and 47.4% in those with cytogenetic relapse), which improved to 70.3% during the entire study period. Overall molecular response (CMR and MMR) was achieved in 97.3% patients (36/37 patients). These excellent molecular results, much better than the ones achieved by front-line use of imatinib in CP CML patients, likely represent the combined effects of GvL and imatinib usage. These investigators also report that of the patients who stopped imatinib in CMR, two-thirds lost CMR, all of whom regained CMR with the reintroduction of imatinib or use of DLI.[117] There was a trend toward longer duration of imatinib treatment in patients with sustained CMR after imatinib discontinuation (269 days) in comparison with those who lost CMR (151 days).

No prospective data compare DLI with imatinib in the relapse setting. In a retrospective review, Weisser and colleagues[118] analyzed outcomes of 31 patients (24 CP, 7 AP) who received DLI (n = 21) or imatinib (n = 10), and reported higher relapse rate with imatinib than with DLI (60% vs 14%, P = .006). However, there was a better OS trend in the imatinib arm, likely due to development of grade II to IV GVHD in 52% and chronic extensive GVHD in 33% of patients in the DLI arm.

Synergism of the combination therapy of DLI and imatinib has also been suggested in a study by Savani and colleagues,[114] in which patients relapsing after allo-SCT were retrospectively analyzed in 4 groups depending on post–allo-SCT therapy received: imatinib alone, DLI alone, concurrent combination therapy, and sequential therapy. Faster molecular responses were reported with the concurrent therapy. In addition, most patients on the imatinib-only arm relapsed after imatinib discontinuation, unlike in the combination arm where the majority of patients maintained the molecular response even after imatinib discontinuation. Prospective evaluation of this approach is needed.

ROLE OF STEM CELL HARVESTING AND AUTOLOGOUS STEM CELL TRANSPLANT

There has been some interest in stem cell collection at the time of CCyR on TKI therapy for potential use at a later time if there is evidence of disease progression. The United Kingdom CML Working Party reported on 58 patients in CCyR using recombinant human granulocyte colony-stimulating factor (G-CSF) while continuing imatinib therapy.[119] Collection goal ($\geq$2 $\times$ 10^6 CD34$^+$ cells/kg body weight) was achieved in 40% patients, all of whom had CML duration of less than 50 months. The median number of apheresis procedures was 2. Apheresis product was negative for Ph chromosome by cytogenetics and fluorescence in situ hybridization in 84% of cases, though the majority had positive Bcr-Abl transcript levels.[119] Hui and colleagues[120] reported that short-term interruption (5–7 days before stem cell collection and until the completion of apheresis) of imatinib improved the CD34$^+$ collection, with 71% achieving the target cell dose (median number of apheresis cycles needed: 1) compared with 50% in the group where imatinib was uninterrupted (median number of apheresis cycle needed: 3). Kreuzer and colleagues[121] performed G-CSF–induced stem cell mobilization during imatinib therapy in 18 patients in CCyR. Apheresis was successful in 72% of patients, with no significant change in PB Bcr-Abl transcript levels after mobilization. Perseghin and colleagues[122] attempted in vivo purging by increasing the imatinib dose to 800 mg daily for 15 days prior to starting G-CSF in 18 patients who had achieved CCyR on imatinib. Of these, 50% failed to mobilize after first apheresis collection. Myelosuppression from high-dose imatinib (as indicated by significantly lower premobilization and day 5 white blood cell count) could have contributed to the poor collection. For the second collection, imatinib was withheld and two-thirds was able to be collected. At the authors' institution, Gordon and colleagues[123] reported on 19 patients who had achieved CCyR on imatinib. Eighty-nine percent achieved target yields without imatinib discontinuation, with the remaining 11% achieving target yield with a brief imatinib discontinuation giving 100% success rate. The majority of patients in this study were being treated with imatinib as front-line therapy, which might have contributed to improved mobilization success rate compared with other reported studies. This study also reported safety with this approach, with all patients remaining in CCyR after a median follow-up of 18 months and none requiring autologous transplant.[123] Bashir and colleagues[124] reported on G-CSF mobilization on 24 patients in CP1 who had achieved CCyR on imatinib. Seventy-three percent achieved the target cell dose (the majority were BM harvest). Stopping imatinib prior to mobilization was associated with significantly higher CD34$^+$ cell yield in this study.[124] In contrast to a relative abundance of data on stem cell collection, there have been only anecdotal reports of patients undergoing autologous transplants in the TKI era.[41,121,124] Current European LeukemiaNet guidelines do not mention autologous transplants or stem cell mobilization/collection.[73] This fact is in line with the clinical practice that most centers do not advocate stem cell mobilization/collection for CML patients.

SUMMARY AND CURRENT RECOMMENDATIONS

In the pre-TKI era, allo-SCT was the front-line treatment of choice for young patients with CML with good performance status. During the initial few years after the introduction of imatinib, there was a debate as to whether TKI therapy should replace allo-SCT

Box 1
Indications for allo-SCT in CML

Blast Phase	Accelerated Phase	First Chronic Phase
As soon as possible after reestablishing CP with TKI or chemotherapy (consider use postengraftment therapy with second-generation TKI)	Less advanced AP at diagnosis—treat as first CP	Failure of second-generation TKI (donor search should be undertaken after failure of imatinib)
	Near BP or evolution into AP on TKI—treat as BP	Imatinib failure and T315I Bcr-Abl1 mutation

Data from Pavlu J, Szydlo RM, Goldman JM, et al. Three decades of transplantation for chronic myeloid leukemia: what have we learnt? Blood 2011;117(3):755–63.

as front-line treatment for all patients, given the lack of randomized data. Now, a decade after the introduction of imatinib, this debate is largely over, with imatinib being well established as front-line therapy with excellent long-term outcomes. For patients with high-risk CML by Sokal/Hasford criteria,[125,126] a case for early transplantation in CP1 could be made, especially if they have low EBMT score or HCT-CI. However, in practical terms this is a small population of individuals and, given the effectiveness of TKIs, unless there are other mitigating factors (such as economic considerations),[49,50] almost all newly diagnosed CML patients are offered TKIs upfront.

Current indications for allo-SCT include patients in AP/BP CML, failure of a second-generation TKIs, and development of TKI-resistant mutations such as T315I. For those with BP or AP, every effort should be made to induce second CP prior to transplant (**Box 1**). The outcomes of URD and MSD transplant are nearly equivalent, but advanced disease continues to negatively affect treatment outcomes. Because many patients are older and heavily pretreated, many centers routinely use RIC regimens, sometimes combined with in vivo T-cell depletion. Some of the best long-term rates of disease control have been achieved with the combination of such regimens and posttransplant treatment of cytogenetic or molecular relapse using TKIs, low-dose DLI, or combinations of the two.

Allo-SCT has a completely different mechanism of action to that of the TKIs. Its effects are to a large extent immunologically mediated and, in contrast to the TKIs, allo-SCT can induce eradication of the leukemic stem cells and cure. Its role in the management of CML will require continual reappraisal as medical therapies continue to evolve.[127]

REFERENCES

1. Druker BJ, Talpaz M, Resta DJ, et al. Efficacy and safety of a specific inhibitor of the BCR-ABL tyrosine kinase in chronic myeloid leukemia. N Engl J Med 2001; 344(14):1031–7.
2. Bjorkholm M, Ohm L, Eloranta S, et al. Success story of targeted therapy in chronic myeloid leukemia: a population-based study of patients diagnosed in Sweden from 1973 to 2008. J Clin Oncol 2011;29(18):2514–20.
3. Fefer A, Buckner CD, Thomas ED, et al. Cure of hematologic neoplasia with transplantation of marrow from identical twins. N Engl J Med 1977;297(3):146–8.
4. Clift RA, Buckner CD, Thomas ED, et al. Treatment of chronic granulocytic leukaemia in chronic phase by allogeneic marrow transplantation. Lancet 1982;2(8299):621–3.
5. Goldman JM, Baughan AS, McCarthy DM, et al. Marrow transplantation for patients in the chronic phase of chronic granulocytic leukaemia. Lancet 1982; 2(8299):623–5.
6. Speck B, Bortin MM, Champlin R, et al. Allogeneic bone-marrow transplantation for chronic myelogenous leukaemia. Lancet 1984;1(8378):665–8.
7. Gratwohl A, Baldomero H, Horisberger B, et al. Current trends in hematopoietic stem cell transplantation in Europe. Blood 2002;100(7):2374–86.
8. Thomas ED, Clift RA, Fefer A, et al. Marrow transplantation for the treatment of chronic myelogenous leukemia. Ann Intern Med 1986;104(2):155–63.
9. Crawley C, Szydlo R, Lalancette M, et al. Outcomes of reduced-intensity transplantation for chronic myeloid leukemia: an analysis of prognostic factors from the Chronic Leukemia Working Party of the EBMT. Blood 2005;106(9):2969–76.
10. Goldman JM, Szydlo R, Horowitz MM, et al. Choice of pretransplant treatment and timing of transplants for chronic myelogenous leukemia in chronic phase. Blood 1993;82(7):2235–8.

11. Robin M, Guardiola P, Devergie A, et al. A 10-year median follow-up study after allogeneic stem cell transplantation for chronic myeloid leukemia in chronic phase from HLA-identical sibling donors. Leukemia 2005;19(9):1613–20.
12. Hansen JA, Gooley TA, Martin PJ, et al. Bone marrow transplants from unrelated donors for patients with chronic myeloid leukemia. N Engl J Med 1998;338(14): 962–8.
13. Goldman JM, Majhail NS, Klein JP, et al. Relapse and late mortality in 5-year survivors of myeloablative allogeneic hematopoietic cell transplantation for chronic myeloid leukemia in first chronic phase. J Clin Oncol 2010;28(11):1888–95.
14. Available at: http://seer.cancer.gov/statfacts/html/cmyl.html. Accessed September 27, 2011.
15. Goldman JM, Gale RP, Horowitz MM, et al. Bone marrow transplantation for chronic myelogenous leukemia in chronic phase. Increased risk for relapse associated with T-cell depletion. Ann Intern Med 1988;108(6):806–14.
16. Marmont AM, Horowitz MM, Gale RP, et al. T-cell depletion of HLA-identical transplants in leukemia. Blood 1991;78(8):2120–30.
17. Buckner CD, Stewart P, Clift RA, et al. Treatment of blastic transformation of chronic granulocytic leukemia by chemotherapy, total body irradiation and infusion of cryopreserved autologous marrow. Exp Hematol 1978;6(1):96–109.
18. Goldman JM, Th'ng KH, Park DS, et al. Collection, cryopreservation and subsequent viability of haemopoietic stem cells intended for treatment of chronic granulocytic leukaemia in blast-cell transformation. Br J Haematol 1978;40(2):185–95.
19. Reiffers J, Trouette R, Marit G, et al. Autologous blood stem cell transplantation for chronic granulocytic leukaemia in transformation: a report of 47 cases. Br J Haematol 1991;77(3):339–45.
20. McGlave PB, De Fabritiis P, Deisseroth A, et al. Autologous transplants for chronic myelogenous leukaemia: results from eight transplant groups. Lancet 1994;343(8911):1486–8.
21. Khouri IF, Kantarjian HM, Talpaz M, et al. Results with high-dose chemotherapy and unpurged autologous stem cell transplantation in 73 patients with chronic myelogenous leukemia: the MD Anderson experience. Bone Marrow Transplant 1996;17(5):775–9.
22. Deisseroth AB, Zu Z, Claxton D, et al. Genetic marking shows that Ph+ cells present in autologous transplants of chronic myelogenous leukemia (CML) contribute to relapse after autologous bone marrow in CML. Blood 1994; 83(10):3068–76.
23. Kolb HJ, Mittermuller J, Clemm C, et al. Donor leukocyte transfusions for treatment of recurrent chronic myelogenous leukemia in marrow transplant patients. Blood 1990;76(12):2462–5.
24. Kolb HJ, Schattenberg A, Goldman JM, et al. Graft-versus-leukemia effect of donor lymphocyte transfusions in marrow grafted patients. Blood 1995;86(5): 2041–50.
25. Collins RH Jr, Shpilberg O, Drobyski WR, et al. Donor leukocyte infusions in 140 patients with relapsed malignancy after allogeneic bone marrow transplantation. J Clin Oncol 1997;15(2):433–44.
26. Dazzi F, Szydlo RM, Cross NC, et al. Durability of responses following donor lymphocyte infusions for patients who relapse after allogeneic stem cell transplantation for chronic myeloid leukemia. Blood 2000;96(8):2712–6.
27. Guglielmi C, Arcese W, Dazzi F, et al. Donor lymphocyte infusion for relapsed chronic myelogenous leukemia: prognostic relevance of the initial cell dose. Blood 2002;100(2):397–405.

28. Weiden PL, Sullivan KM, Flournoy N, et al. Antileukemic effect of chronic graft-versus-host disease: contribution to improved survival after allogeneic marrow transplantation. N Engl J Med 1981;304(25):1529–33.
29. Horowitz MM, Gale RP, Sondel PM, et al. Graft-versus-leukemia reactions after bone marrow transplantation. Blood 1990;75(3):555–62.
30. Slavin S, Naparstek E, Nagler A, et al. Allogeneic cell therapy for relapsed leukemia after bone marrow transplantation with donor peripheral blood lymphocytes. Exp Hematol 1995;23(14):1553–62.
31. Giralt S, Estey E, Albitar M, et al. Engraftment of allogeneic hematopoietic progenitor cells with purine analog-containing chemotherapy: harnessing graft-versus-leukaemia without myeloablative therapy. Blood 1997;89(12):4531–6.
32. Childs R, Epperson D, Bahceci E, et al. Molecular remission of chronic myeloid leukaemia following a non-myeloablative allogeneic peripheral blood stem cell transplant: in vivo and in vitro evidence for a graft-versus-leukaemia effect. Br J Haematol 1999;107(2):396–400.
33. McSweeney PA, Niederwieser D, Shizuru JA, et al. Hematopoietic cell transplantation in older patients with hematologic malignancies: replacing high-dose cytotoxic therapy with graft-versus-tumor effects. Blood 2001;97(11):3390–400.
34. Das M, Saikia TK, Advani SH, et al. Use of a reduced-intensity conditioning regimen for allogeneic transplantation in patients with chronic myeloid leukemia. Bone Marrow Transplant 2003;32(2):125–9.
35. Or R, Shapira MY, Resnick I, et al. Nonmyeloablative allogeneic stem cell transplantation for the treatment of chronic myeloid leukemia in first chronic phase. Blood 2003;101(2):441–5.
36. Weisser M, Schleuning M, Ledderose G, et al. Reduced-intensity conditioning using TBI (8 Gy), fludarabine, cyclophosphamide and ATG in elderly CML patients provides excellent results especially when performed in the early course of the disease. Bone Marrow Transplant 2004;34(12):1083–8.
37. Kerbauy FR, Storb R, Hegenbart U, et al. Hematopoietic cell transplantation from HLA-identical sibling donors after low-dose radiation-based conditioning for treatment of CML. Leukemia 2005;19(6):990–7.
38. Kebriaei P, Detry MA, Giralt S, et al. Long-term follow-up of allogeneic hematopoietic stem-cell transplantation with reduced-intensity conditioning for patients with chronic myeloid leukemia. Blood 2007;110(9):3456–62.
39. Champlin R, de Lima M, Kebriaei P, et al. Nonmyeloablative allogeneic stem cell transplantation for chronic myelogenous leukemia in the imatinib era. Clin Lymphoma Myeloma 2009;9(Suppl 3):S261–5.
40. Slavin S, Nagler A, Naparstek E, et al. Nonmyeloablative stem cell transplantation and cell therapy as an alternative to conventional bone marrow transplantation with lethal cytoreduction for the treatment of malignant and nonmalignant hematologic diseases. Blood 1998;91(3):756–63.
41. Luo Y, Lai XY, Tan YM, et al. Reduced-intensity allogeneic transplantation combined with imatinib mesylate for chronic myeloid leukemia in first chronic phase. Leukemia 2009;23(6):1171–4.
42. Poire X, Artz A, Larson RA, et al. Allogeneic stem cell transplantation with alemtuzumab-based conditioning for patients with advanced chronic myelogenous leukemia. Leuk Lymphoma 2009;50(1):85–91.
43. Raiola AM, Van Lint MT, Lamparelli T, et al. Reduced intensity thiotepa-cyclophosphamide conditioning for allogeneic haemopoietic stem cell transplants (HSCT) in patients up to 60 years of age. Br J Haematol 2000;109(4):716–21.

44. Bornhauser M, Kiehl M, Siegert W, et al. Dose-reduced conditioning for allografting in 44 patients with chronic myeloid leukaemia: a retrospective analysis. Br J Haematol 2001;115(1):119–24.

45. Gratwohl A, Brand R, Apperley J, et al. Allogeneic hematopoietic stem cell transplantation for chronic myeloid leukemia in Europe 2006: transplant activity, long-term data and current results. An analysis by the Chronic Leukemia Working Party of the European Group for Blood and Marrow Transplantation (EBMT). Haematologica 2006;91(4):513–21.

46. Gratwohl A, Heim D. Current role of stem cell transplantation in chronic myeloid leukaemia. Best Pract Res Clin Haematol 2009;22(3):431–43.

47. Bacher U, Klyuchnikov E, Zabelina T, et al. The changing scene of allogeneic stem cell transplantation for chronic myeloid leukemia—a report from the German Registry covering the period from 1998 to 2004. Ann Hematol 2009; 88(12):1237–47.

48. Giralt SA, Arora M, Goldman JM, et al. Impact of imatinib therapy on the use of allogeneic haematopoietic progenitor cell transplantation for the treatment of chronic myeloid leukaemia. Br J Haematol 2007;137(5):461–7.

49. Ruiz-Argüelles GJ, Gomez-Almaguer D, Morales-Toquero A, et al. The early referral for reduced-intensity stem cell transplantation in patients with Ph1 (+) chronic myelogenous leukemia in chronic phase in the imatinib era: results of the Latin American Cooperative Oncohematology Group (LACOHG) prospective, multicenter study. Bone Marrow Transplant 2005;36(12):1043–7.

50. Gratwohl A, Baldomero H, Schwendener A, et al. Hematopoietic stem cell transplants for chronic myeloid leukemia in Europe—impact of cost considerations. Leukemia 2007;21(3):383–6.

51. Hehlmann R, Berger U, Pfirrmann M, et al. Drug treatment is superior to allografting as first-line therapy in chronic myeloid leukemia. Blood 2007;109(11): 4686–92.

52. Bittencourt H, Funke V, Fogliatto L, et al. Imatinib mesylate versus allogeneic BMT for patients with chronic myeloid leukemia in first chronic phase. Bone Marrow Transplant 2008;42(9):597–600.

53. Saussele S, Lauseker M, Gratwohl A, et al. Allogeneic hematopoietic stem cell transplantation (allo SCT) for chronic myeloid leukemia in the imatinib era: evaluation of its impact within a subgroup of the randomized German CML Study IV. Blood 2010;115(10):1880–5.

54. Cwynarski K, Roberts IA, Iacobelli S, et al. Stem cell transplantation for chronic myeloid leukemia in children. Blood 2003;102(4):1224–31.

55. Suttorp M, Claviez A, Bader P, et al. Allogeneic stem cell transplantation for pediatric and adolescent patients with CML: results from the prospective trial CML-paed I. Klin Padiatr 2009;221(6):351–7.

56. Apperley J. CML in pregnancy and childhood. Best Pract Res Clin Haematol 2009;22(3):455–74.

57. Palandri F, Castagnetti F, Testoni N, et al. Chronic myeloid leukemia in blast crisis treated with imatinib 600 mg: outcome of the patients alive after a 6-year follow-up. Haematologica 2008;93(12):1792–6.

58. Palandri F, Castagnetti F, Alimena G, et al. The long-term durability of cytogenetic responses in patients with accelerated phase chronic myeloid leukemia treated with imatinib 600 mg: the GIMEMA CML Working Party experience after a 7-year follow-up. Haematologica 2009;94(2):205–12.

59. Silver RT, Cortes J, Waltzman R, et al. Sustained durability of responses and improved progression-free and overall survival with imatinib treatment for

accelerated phase and blast crisis chronic myeloid leukemia: long-term follow-up of the STI571 0102 and 0109 trials. Haematologica 2009;94(5):743–4.

60. Jiang Q, Xu LP, Liu DH, et al. Imatinib mesylate versus allogeneic hematopoietic stem cell transplantation for patients with chronic myelogenous leukemia in the accelerated phase. Blood 2011;117(11):3032–40.

61. Deininger M, Schleuning M, Greinix H, et al. The effect of prior exposure to imatinib on transplant-related mortality. Haematologica 2006;91(4):452–9.

62. Lee SJ, Kukreja M, Wang T, et al. Impact of prior imatinib mesylate on the outcome of hematopoietic cell transplantation for chronic myeloid leukemia. Blood 2008;112(8):3500–7.

63. Shimoni A, Kroger N, Zander AR, et al. Imatinib mesylate (STI571) in preparation for allogeneic hematopoietic stem cell transplantation and donor lymphocyte infusions in patients with Philadelphia-positive acute leukemias. Leukemia 2003;17(2):290–7.

64. Zaucha JM, Prejzner W, Giebel S, et al. Imatinib therapy prior to myeloablative allogeneic stem cell transplantation. Bone Marrow Transplant 2005;36(5):417–24.

65. Oehler VG, Gooley T, Snyder DS, et al. The effects of imatinib mesylate treatment before allogeneic transplantation for chronic myeloid leukemia. Blood 2007;109(4):1782–9.

66. Hehlmann R, Hochhaus A, Baccarani M. Chronic myeloid leukaemia. Lancet 2007;370(9584):342–50.

67. Brave M, Goodman V, Kaminskas E, et al. Sprycel for chronic myeloid leukemia and Philadelphia chromosome-positive acute lymphoblastic leukemia resistant to or intolerant of imatinib mesylate. Clin Cancer Res 2008;14(2):352–9.

68. Hazarika M, Jiang X, Liu Q, et al. Tasigna for chronic and accelerated phase Philadelphia chromosome—positive chronic myelogenous leukemia resistant to or intolerant of imatinib. Clin Cancer Res 2008;14(17):5325–31.

69. Kantarjian H, Shah NP, Hochhaus A, et al. Dasatinib versus imatinib in newly diagnosed chronic-phase chronic myeloid leukemia. N Engl J Med 2010;362(24):2260–70.

70. Saglio G, Kim DW, Issaragrisil S, et al. Nilotinib versus imatinib for newly diagnosed chronic myeloid leukemia. N Engl J Med 2010;362(24):2251–9.

71. Jabbour E, Cortes J, Kantarjian H, et al. Novel tyrosine kinase inhibitor therapy before allogeneic stem cell transplantation in patients with chronic myeloid leukemia: no evidence for increased transplant-related toxicity. Cancer 2007;110(2):340–4.

72. Shimoni A, Leiba M, Schleuning M, et al. Prior treatment with the tyrosine kinase inhibitors dasatinib and nilotinib allows stem cell transplantation (SCT) in a less advanced disease phase and does not increase SCT toxicity in patients with chronic myelogenous leukemia and Philadelphia positive acute lymphoblastic leukemia. Leukemia 2009;23(1):190–4.

73. Baccarani M, Cortes J, Pane F, et al. Chronic myeloid leukemia: an update of concepts and management recommendations of European LeukemiaNet. J Clin Oncol 2009;27(35):6041–51.

74. Velev N, Cortes J, Champlin R, et al. Stem cell transplantation for patients with chronic myeloid leukemia resistant to tyrosine kinase inhibitors with BCR-ABL kinase domain mutation T315I. Cancer 2010;116(15):3631–7.

75. Basak G, Torosian T, Snarski E, et al. Hematopoietic stem cell transplantation for T315I-mutated chronic myelogenous leukemia. Ann Transplant 2010;15(2):68–70.

76. Sanchez-Guijo FM, Lopez-Jimenez J, Gonzalez T, et al. Multitargeted sequential therapy with MK-0457 and dasatinib followed by stem cell transplantation for T315I mutated chronic myeloid leukemia. Leuk Res 2009;33(6):e20–2.

77. Jabbour E, Cortes J, Santos FP, et al. Results of allogeneic hematopoietic stem cell transplantation for chronic myelogenous leukemia patients who failed tyrosine kinase inhibitors after developing BCR-ABL1 kinase domain mutations. Blood 2011;117(13):3641–7.

78. Nicolini FE, Basak GW, Soverini S, et al. Allogeneic stem cell transplantation for patients harboring T315I BCR-ABL mutated leukemias. Blood 2011. [Epub ahead of print].

79. Nicolini FE, Mauro MJ, Martinelli G, et al. Epidemiologic study on survival of chronic myeloid leukemia and Ph(+) acute lymphoblastic leukemia patients with BCR-ABL T315I mutation. Blood;114(26):5271–8.

80. Cortes J, Talpaz M, Bixby D, et al. A phase 1 trial of oral Ponatinib (AP24534) in patients with refractory chronic myelogenous leukemia (CML) and other hematologic malignancies: emerging safety and clinical response findings. Blood 2010;116:210.

81. Gratwohl A, Hermans J, Goldman JM, et al. Risk assessment for patients with chronic myeloid leukaemia before allogeneic blood or marrow transplantation. Chronic Leukemia Working Party of the European Group for Blood and Marrow Transplantation. Lancet 1998;352(9134):1087–92.

82. Passweg JR, Walker I, Sobocinski KA, et al. Validation and extension of the EBMT Risk Score for patients with chronic myeloid leukaemia (CML) receiving allogeneic haematopoietic stem cell transplants. Br J Haematol 2004;125(5):613–20.

83. Pavlu J, Kew AK, Taylor-Roberts B, et al. Optimizing patient selection for myeloablative allogeneic hematopoietic cell transplantation in chronic myeloid leukemia in chronic phase. Blood 2010;115(20):4018–20.

84. Artz AS, Wickrema A, Dinner S, et al. Pretreatment C-reactive protein is a predictor for outcomes after reduced-intensity allogeneic hematopoietic cell transplantation. Biol Blood Marrow Transplant 2008;14(11):1209–16.

85. Elmaagacli AH, Beelen DW, Opalka B, et al. The risk of residual molecular and cytogenetic disease in patients with Philadelphia-chromosome positive first chronic phase chronic myelogenous leukemia is reduced after transplantation of allogeneic peripheral blood stem cells compared with bone marrow. Blood 1999;94(2):384–9.

86. Stem Cell Trialists' Collaborative Group. Allogeneic peripheral blood stem-cell compared with bone marrow transplantation in the management of hematologic malignancies: an individual patient data meta-analysis of nine randomized trials. J Clin Oncol 2005;23(22):5074–87.

87. Eapen M, Logan BR, Confer DL, et al. Peripheral blood grafts from unrelated donors are associated with increased acute and chronic graft-versus-host disease without improved survival. Biol Blood Marrow Transplant 2007;13(12):1461–8.

88. Champlin RE, Schmitz N, Horowitz MM, et al. Blood stem cells compared with bone marrow as a source of hematopoietic cells for allogeneic transplantation. IBMTR Histocompatibility and Stem Cell Sources Working Committee and the European Group for Blood and Marrow Transplantation (EBMT). Blood 2000; 95(12):3702–9.

89. Schmitz N, Eapen M, Horowitz MM, et al. Long-term outcome of patients given transplants of mobilized blood or bone marrow: a report from the International Bone Marrow Transplant Registry and the European Group for Blood and Marrow Transplantation. Blood 2006;108(13):4288–90.

90. Oehler VG, Radich JP, Storer B, et al. Randomized trial of allogeneic related bone marrow transplantation versus peripheral blood stem cell transplantation for chronic myeloid leukemia. Biol Blood Marrow Transplant 2005;11(2):85–92.

91. Weisdorf DJ, Anasetti C, Antin JH, et al. Allogeneic bone marrow transplantation for chronic myelogenous leukemia: comparative analysis of unrelated versus matched sibling donor transplantation. Blood 2002;99(6):1971–7.

92. Arora M, Weisdorf DJ, Spellman SR, et al. HLA-identical sibling compared with 8/8 matched and mismatched unrelated donor bone marrow transplant for chronic phase chronic myeloid leukemia. J Clin Oncol 2009;27(10):1644–52.

93. Sanz J, Montesinos P, Saavedra S, et al. Single-unit umbilical cord blood transplantation from unrelated donors in adult patients with chronic myelogenous leukemia. Biol Blood Marrow Transplant 2010;16(11):1589–95.

94. Nagamura-Inoue T, Kai S, Azuma H, et al. Unrelated cord blood transplantation in CML: Japan Cord Blood Bank Network analysis. Bone Marrow Transplant 2008;42(4):241–51.

95. Socie G, Clift RA, Blaise D, et al. Busulfan plus cyclophosphamide compared with total-body irradiation plus cyclophosphamide before marrow transplantation for myeloid leukemia: long-term follow-up of 4 randomized studies. Blood 2001;98(13):3569–74.

96. Andersson BS, Thall PF, Madden T, et al. Busulfan systemic exposure relative to regimen-related toxicity and acute graft-versus-host disease: defining a therapeutic window for i.v. BuCy2 in chronic myelogenous leukemia. Biol Blood Marrow Transplant 2002;8(9):477–85.

97. Radich JP, Gooley T, Bensinger W, et al. HLA-matched related hematopoietic cell transplantation for chronic-phase CML using a targeted busulfan and cyclophosphamide preparative regimen. Blood 2003;102(1):31–5.

98. Olavarria E, Siddique S, Griffiths MJ, et al. Posttransplantation imatinib as a strategy to postpone the requirement for immunotherapy in patients undergoing reduced-intensity allografts for chronic myeloid leukemia. Blood 2007;110(13):4614–7.

99. Chakrabarti S, MacDonald D, Hale G, et al. T-cell depletion with Campath-1H "in the bag" for matched related allogeneic peripheral blood stem cell transplantation is associated with reduced graft-versus-host disease, rapid immune constitution and improved survival. Br J Haematol 2003;121(1):109–18.

100. von dem Borne PA, Beaumont F, Starrenburg CW, et al. Outcomes after myeloablative unrelated donor stem cell transplantation using both in vitro and in vivo T-cell depletion with alemtuzumab. Haematologica 2006;91(11):1559–62.

101. Holowiecki J, Giebel S, Wojnar J, et al. Treosulfan and fludarabine low-toxicity conditioning for allogeneic haematopoietic stem cell transplantation in chronic myeloid leukaemia. Br J Haematol 2008;142(2):284–92.

102. Hughes TP, Morgan GJ, Martiat P, et al. Detection of residual leukemia after bone marrow transplant for chronic myeloid leukemia: role of polymerase chain reaction in predicting relapse. Blood 1991;77(4):874–8.

103. Lin F, van Rhee F, Goldman JM, et al. Kinetics of increasing BCR-ABL transcript numbers in chronic myeloid leukemia patients who relapse after bone marrow transplantation. Blood 1996;87(10):4473–8.

104. Radich JP, Gehly G, Gooley T, et al. Polymerase chain reaction detection of the BCR-ABL fusion transcript after allogeneic marrow transplantation for chronic myeloid leukemia: results and implications in 346 patients. Blood 1995;85(9):2632–8.

105. Kaeda J, O'Shea D, Szydlo RM, et al. Serial measurement of BCR-ABL transcripts in the peripheral blood after allogeneic stem cell transplantation for

chronic myeloid leukemia: an attempt to define patients who may not require further therapy. Blood 2006;107(10):4171–6.

106. Olavarria E, Kanfer E, Szydlo R, et al. Early detection of BCR-ABL transcripts by quantitative reverse transcriptase-polymerase chain reaction predicts outcome after allogeneic stem cell transplantation for chronic myeloid leukemia. Blood 2001;97(6):1560–5.

107. White HE, Matejtschuk P, Rigsby P, et al. Establishment of the 1st World Health Organization International Genetic Reference Panel for quantitation of BCR-ABL mRNA. Blood 2010;116(22):e111–7.

108. Mackinnon S, Papadopoulos EB, Carabasi MH, et al. Adoptive immunotherapy evaluating escalating doses of donor leukocytes for relapse of chronic myeloid leukemia after bone marrow transplantation: separation of graft-versus-leukemia responses from graft-versus-host disease. Blood 1995;86(4):1261–8.

109. Dazzi F, Szydlo RM, Craddock C, et al. Comparison of single-dose and escalating-dose regimens of donor lymphocyte infusion for relapse after allografting for chronic myeloid leukemia. Blood 2000;95(1):67–71.

110. Chalandon Y, Passweg JR, Schmid C, et al. Outcome of patients developing GVHD after DLI given to treat CML relapse: a study by the Chronic Leukemia Working Party of the EBMT. Bone Marrow Transplant 2010;45(3):558–64.

111. Craddock C, Szydlo RM, Klein JP, et al. Estimating leukemia-free survival after allografting for chronic myeloid leukemia: a new method that takes into account patients who relapse and are restored to complete remission. Blood 2000;96(1): 86–90.

112. Carpenter PA, Snyder DS, Flowers ME, et al. Prophylactic administration of imatinib after hematopoietic cell transplantation for high-risk Philadelphia chromosome-positive leukemia. Blood 2007;109(7):2791–3.

113. Sillaber C, Herrmann H, Bennett K, et al. Immunosuppression and atypical infections in CML patients treated with dasatinib at 140 mg daily. Eur J Clin Invest 2009;39(12):1098–109.

114. Savani BN, Montero A, Kurlander R, et al. Imatinib synergizes with donor lymphocyte infusions to achieve rapid molecular remission of CML relapsing after allogeneic stem cell transplantation. Bone Marrow Transplant 2005; 36(11):1009–15.

115. Kantarjian HM, O'Brien S, Cortes JE, et al. Imatinib mesylate therapy for relapse after allogeneic stem cell transplantation for chronic myelogenous leukemia. Blood 2002;100(5):1590–5.

116. Olavarria E, Ottmann OG, Deininger M, et al. Response to imatinib in patients who relapse after allogeneic stem cell transplantation for chronic myeloid leukemia. Leukemia 2003;17(9):1707–12.

117. Hess G, Bunjes D, Siegert W, et al. Sustained complete molecular remissions after treatment with imatinib-mesylate in patients with failure after allogeneic stem cell transplantation for chronic myelogenous leukemia: results of a prospective phase II open-label multicenter study. J Clin Oncol 2005;23(30):7583–93.

118. Weisser M, Tischer J, Schnittger S, et al. A comparison of donor lymphocyte infusions or imatinib mesylate for patients with chronic myelogenous leukemia who have relapsed after allogeneic stem cell transplantation. Haematologica 2006;91(5):663–6.

119. Drummond MW, Marin D, Clark RE, et al. Mobilization of Ph chromosome-negative peripheral blood stem cells in chronic myeloid leukaemia patients with imatinib mesylate-induced complete cytogenetic remission. Br J Haematol 2003;123(3):479–83.

120. Hui CH, Goh KY, White D, et al. Successful peripheral blood stem cell mobilisation with filgrastim in patients with chronic myeloid leukaemia achieving complete cytogenetic response with imatinib, without increasing disease burden as measured by quantitative real-time PCR. Leukemia 2003;17(5):821–8.

121. Kreuzer KA, Kluhs C, Baskaynak G, et al. Filgrastim-induced stem cell mobilization in chronic myeloid leukaemia patients during imatinib therapy: safety, feasibility and evidence for an efficient in vivo purging. Br J Haematol 2004;124(2): 195–9.

122. Perseghin P, Gambacorti-Passerini C, Tornaghi L, et al. Peripheral blood progenitor cell collection in chronic myeloid leukemia patients with complete cytogenetic response after treatment with imatinib mesylate. Transfusion 2005; 45(7):1214–20.

123. Gordon MK, Sher D, Karrison T, et al. Successful autologous stem cell collection in patients with chronic myeloid leukemia in complete cytogenetic response, with quantitative measurement of BCR-ABL expression in blood, marrow, and apheresis products. Leuk Lymphoma 2008;49(3):531–7.

124. Bashir Q, De Lima MJ, McMannis JD, et al. Hematopoietic progenitor cell collection in patients with chronic myelogenous leukemia in complete cytogenetic remission after imatinib mesylate therapy. Leuk Lymphoma 2010;51(8):1478–84.

125. Sokal JE, Cox EB, Baccarani M, et al. Prognostic discrimination in "good-risk" chronic granulocytic leukemia. Blood 1984;63(4):789–99.

126. Hasford J, Pfirrmann M, Hehlmann R, et al. A new prognostic score for survival of patients with chronic myeloid leukemia treated with interferon alfa. Writing Committee for the Collaborative CML Prognostic Factors Project Group. J Natl Cancer Inst 1998;90(11):850–8.

127. Pavlu J, Szydlo RM, Goldman JM, et al. Three decades of transplantation for chronic myeloid leukemia: what have we learnt? Blood 2011;117(3):755–63.

Portal Vein Thrombosis and Budd–Chiari Syndrome

Paulo Lisboa Bittencourt, MD, PhD[a],*,
Cláudia Alves Couto, MD, PhD[b], Daniel Dias Ribeiro, MD, PhD[b,c]

KEYWORDS
- Portal vein thrombosis • Budd–Chiari syndrome • Cirrhosis
- Thrombophilia • Portal hypertension

Portal vein thrombosis (PVT) and Budd–Chiari syndrome (BCS) are caused by thrombosis and/or obstruction of the extrahepatic portal veins and the hepatic venous outflow tract, respectively.[1–3] Several heterogeneous prothrombotic disorders may cause thrombosis of the portal and hepatic veins.[2,3] Venous thrombosis usually results from the convergence of vessel wall injury and/or venous stasis, known as local triggering factors, and the occurrence of acquired and/or inherited thrombophilia, also known as systemic prothrombotic risk factors.[4–6]

RISK FACTORS FOR PORTAL VEIN THROMBOSIS AND BUDD–CHIARI SYNDROME

Local risk factors are responsible for 30% to 40% of the cases of PVT, but they are rarely reported in subjects with primary BCS.[6,7] Inflammatory intra-abdominal disorders such as appendicitis and pancreatitis, postoperative complications of abdominal surgery, particularly splenectomy and surgical portosystemic shunts, and portal hypertension are recognized intra-abdominal risk factors for PVT (**Table 1**). In contrast, distinct *systemic prothrombotic risk* factors have been recognized in 60% to 70% of PVT and up to 90% of BCS (**Table 2**). All of these have been associated

---

A version of this article originally appeared in *Clinics in Liver Disease*, 13:1.
[a] Unit of Gastroenterology and Hepatology, Portuguese Hospital, Salvador, Bahia, Brazil
[b] Alfa Gastroenterology Institute, Federal University of Minas Gerais, Belo Horizonte, Minas Gerais, Brazil
[c] Department of Hematology, Federal University of Minas Gerais, Belo Horizonte, Minas Gerais, Brazil
* Corresponding author. Rua Prof. Clementino Fraga 220/1901, Salvador, Bahia, Brazil, CEP 40170050.
E-mail address: plbbr@uol.com.br

Hematol Oncol Clin N Am 25 (2011) 1049–1066
doi:10.1016/j.hoc.2011.09.011
0889-8588/11/$ – see front matter © 2011 Elsevier Inc. All rights reserved.

hemonc.theclinics.com

Table 1
Local risk factors associated with portal vein thrombosis and Budd–Chiari syndrome

Portal Vein Thrombosis	Budd–Chiari Syndrome
Focal inflammatory lesions: neonatal omphalitis, diverticulitis, appendicitis, pancreatitis, duodenal ulcer, cholecystitis, tuberculous lymphadenitis, Crohn's disease, ulcerative colitis, cytomegalovirus hepatitis Injury to the portal venous system: splenectomy, colectomy, gastrectomy, cholecystectomy, liver transplantation, abdominal trauma, surgical portosystemic shunting, transjugular intrahepatic portosystemic shunt placement, cirrhosis	Invasion or encasement of inferior vena cava or hepatic veins by neoplasia, liver cysts, or abscess. Budd–Chiari syndrome in this setting can be designated as "secondary" to a local extrinsic factor such as neoplasm, cyst, or abscess, which causes external compression

Adapted from Valla DC. The diagnosis and management of the Budd–Chiari syndrome: consensus and controversies. Hepatology 2003;38:793–803; and Janssen HL, Garcia-Pagan JC, Elias E, et al. Budd–Chiari syndrome: a review by an expert panel. J Hepatol 2003;38:364–71.

Table 2
Frequency of acquired and inherited systemic prothrombotic risk factors in patients with PVT, BCS, DVT, and healthy controls

Prothrombotic Disorders	PVT, %[a]	BCS, %[b]	DVT, %[c]	Healthy Subjects, %[c]
Myeloproliferative diseases[d]	14–35	28–47	NA	NA
Antiphospholipid syndrome	5–23	5–21	4–21	5
Factor V Leiden mutation	3–14	14–31	15–20	5–12
Factor II gene mutation	3–22	4–6	4–8	1
Protein C deficiency	0–9	0–13	3–6	0.2–0.5
Protein S deficiency	2–30	0–6	2	0.03–0.13
Antithrombin deficiency	0–4.5	0–4	0.5–7.5	0.02
C677T MTHFR gene mutations[e]	0–11	13–52	Variable	12–46
Hyperhomocysteinemia	NA	0–37	10–25	5–10
Elevated factor VIII	NA	NA	15–25	NA
Pregnancy	0–4	0–15	[f]	NA
Oral contraceptive use	0–48	7–55	[f]	NA
None	16–22	6–23	50	NA

Several patients had one or more overlapping prothrombotic risk factors.

Abbreviations: BCS, Budd–Chiari syndrome; DVT, deep vein thrombosis; MTHFR, methylene tetrahydrofolate reductase; NA, not applicable; PVT, portal vein thrombosis.

  [a] *Adapted from* Refs.[8–11,53,57]
  [b] *Adapted from* Refs.[9,10,12–15,36]
  [c] *Adapted from* Refs.[4,5,17]
  [d] Occult MPD was not investigated in most of the cohorts.
  [e] The presence of C677T MTHFR gene mutations without an increase in homocystein level is not a risk factor for DVT.
  [f] Accounts for a threefold increase in the relative risk for DVT.

with an increased systemic predisposition to deep vein thrombosis and/or pulmonary embolism and more than one prothrombotic risk factor has been implicated in the pathogenesis of PVT and BCS in up to one third of the patients.[4,5,8–18]

Some risk factors are more frequently associated with one or another of those vascular disorders of the liver. In this respect, most of the cases of PVT are attributable to Philadelphia (Ph) chromosome negative myeloproliferative diseases (MPD), antiphospholipid syndrome, or distinct inherited prothrombotic disorders, such as protein S deficiency and prothrombin gene mutation (see **Table 2**).[7–10] There is a great geographic variation, but MPD is one of the most frequent disorders associated with PVT. In general, the prevalence of inherited thrombophilia is far less common in the East when compared with the West.[11,19,20]

Local risk factors account for only a small number of the cases of BCS, which can then be designated as "secondary" BCS (see **Table 1**). Most patients with BCS have a "primary" disorder and share one or more prothrombotic risk factors, mainly MPD, oral contraceptive use, factor V Leiden mutation, and antiphospholipid syndrome. Myeloproliferative disorders, particularly polycythemia vera, are observed in approximately half of the cases of BCS, but fewer than 10% of the subjects with overt MPD develop BCS.[13] There is also some geographic variation in the prevalence of acquired thrombophilia in patients with BCS. The use of oral contraceptives is related to BCS more frequently in Western, when compared with Eastern patients. On the other hand, poor sanitation has been associated with BCS, particularly with inferior vena cava (IVC) involvement in the Asian countries and poor socioeconomic status.[21]

EVALUATION OF THROMBOPHILIA, PORTAL VEIN THROMBOSIS, AND BUDD–CHIARI SYNDROME

Because of the high frequency of inherited and/or acquired prothrombotic disorders in patients with PVT and BCS, a systematic investigation of these risk factors is warranted and a formal hematological consultation is usually recomended, because the usual diagnostic criteria for those disorders cannot always be applied to subjects with underlying liver disease.[4,18,22,23]

Myeloproliferative diseases are the single most common group of disorders associated with PVT and BCS. In most cases, the Ph chromosome negative MPD can be classified as polycythemia vera, essential thrombocythemia or myelofibrosis. These diagnoses in patients with PVT and BCS, using the current World Health Organization criteria, may be misleading because of the presence of increased plasma volume and hypersplenism in the subjects with chronic liver disease (CLD) and portal hypertension. In this regard, detection of spontaneous endogenous erythrocyte colonies (EEC), determination of the somatic JAK2 V617F mutation,[13,24–27] and bone marrow biopsy to assess the presence of dystrophic megakariocytes has been used to diagnose MPD without typical phenotypic markers in subjects with and without CLD.[8,26] Based on the results of these assays, up to two thirds of the patients with either PVT or BCS were shown to have either overt or occult MPD.[28] However, some drawbacks associated with use of these parameters to diagnose occult MPD have to be highlighted.

The EEC assay is a nonstandardized labor-intensive method that is highly dependant on local laboratory expertise. It can yield negative results in subjects with clear-cut criteria for MPD and positive results in healthy subjects and patients with nonclonal polycythemia,[29] which limits its diagnostic accuracy for MPD.[29–32]

Recently, several investigators have identified an acquired mutation in the autoregulatory pseudokinase domain (JH2) of Janus kinase-2 (JAK2) gene in patients with MPD. One substitution of valine to phenylalanine at position 617 (V617F) was observed in 90% to 95% of the patients with polycythemia vera, 50% to 70% of the patients with essential thrombocythemia, and 40% to 50% of the patients with myelofibrosis.[33] Preliminary data have also suggested that MPD patients with JAK2 have an increased risk of thrombosis, hemorrhage, fibrosis, and cytoreductive treatment requirement when compared with their JAK2 negative counterparts[34]; however, data on the functional consequences of this mutation are still scarce. Noninvasive assessment of V617F JAK2 mutation for evaluation of MPD in patients with hepatic or splanchnic vein thrombosis is promising, but it should be emphasized that its presence is not sufficient for defining the MPD phenotype[23] and that V617F JAK2 mutation may be absent in a significant proportion of patients with PVT and BCS with overt MPD.[35,36]

Antiphospholipid antibodies syndrome (APS) is seen in 5% to 23% of the patients with PVT or BCS. The antiphospholipid antibodies are a group of autoantibodies that target phospholipid binding proteins, including lupus anticoagulant, IgM and IgG anticardiolipin, and antiβ2-glicoprotein I antibodies. As the presence of low-titer anticardiolipin is frequent in subjects with CLD, the diagnostic criteria for APS in such patients requires, apart from past evidence of thrombosis or miscarriages, the detection of one of those antibodies in medium or high titers two times at least 12 weeks apart.[17,37,38]

Inherited deficiencies of antithrombin and proteins S and C are responsible for 15% to 30% of the cases of PVT and BCS. However, their diagnoses are sometimes challenging in patients with liver disease, because low protein levels could be a result of impaired hepatic synthesis and not related to inherited deficiency. In accordance with this assumption is the reversal of coagulation factor abnormalities after surgical treatment of extrahepatic portal vein obstruction (EHPVO) by mesenteric to left portal vein bypass.[39] In practice, deficiency of proteins S and C and antithrombin are assumed when no other abnormality in the coagulation factors levels is disclosed, indicating preserved liver function. Family studies could also be useful in doubtful cases.[13]

Several other divergent situations deserve mention in this section. Increased levels of factor VIII have also been described in patients with BCS and PVT.[2–5] However, as factor VIII is an acute phase protein, its increase could reflect liver disease per se and not inherited thrombophilia. Diagnosis has to rely on the determination of factor VIII levels as well as other acute phase proteins in different time points. Family studies could also be useful in this situation. In contrast, prothrombin G20210A gene mutation and factor V G1691A gene variant are frequently encountered in this setting. Their diagnosis is straightforward based on polymerase chain reaction (PCR)-based assays.[4,5] However, the role of high homocysteine levels in thrombosis is controversial. Hyperhomocysteinemia can be detected by high performance liquid chromatography or chemiluminescence. Testing solely for methylene tetrahydrofolate reductase (MTHFR) C677T gene mutation is unreliable since heterozygosity and homozygosity for MTHFR C677T variant is observed in 50% and 10% of the healthy population, respectively.[4,5] Paroxysmal nocturnal hemoglobinuria and Behcet's disease may also be observed, particularly in subjects with BCS.[2,7,40]

Based on recommendations from an expert panel, the investigation of thrombophilia in patients with BCS and PVT should initially include complete blood cell count, assays for plasma levels of coagulation factors and inhibitors, determination of genetic factor V and prothrombin gene mutations, assessment of antiphospholipid antibodies and lupus anticoagulant, and flow cytometry testing for paroxysmal nocturnal hemoglobinuria. Bone marrow biopsy, determination of blood cell mass and serum erythropoietin, as well as EEC, and the recently discovered JAK2 mutation should be the next steps in the evaluation of MPD (**Table 3**).[2,3,7]

Table 3
Approach to the investigation of acquired and/or inherited thrombophilia in patients with BCS and EHPVO

Myeloproliferative disorders	Complete blood cell count Bone marrow biopsy Determination of total red cell mass and serum erythropoietin after correction for iron deficiency EEC and JAK2 mutation (whether available)
Paroxysmal nocturnal hemoglobinuria	Flow cytometry for CD55- and CD59-deficient cells
Antiphospholipid syndrome	Lupus anticoagulant,[a] IgM and IgG anticardiolipin antibodies, antib2-glicoprotein I and antinuclear factors
Factor V Leiden mutation	Detection of G1691A gene variant by PCR-based methods
Prothrombin gene mutation	Detection of G20210A gene mutation by PCR-based methods
Protein C, S, and Antithrombin III	Functional assays in the presence of normal clotting factor levels plasma levels[a]
Hyperhomocysteinemia	Blood folate, vitamin BI2 and homocysteine levels. Search for MTHFR polymorphism only when the level of homocysteine is high

Abbreviations: BCS, Budd–Chiari syndrome; EEC, endogenous erythrocyte colonies; EHPVO, extrahepatic portal vein obstruction; JAK2, Janus kinase-2; MTHFR, methylene tetrahydrofolate reductase; PCR, polymerase chain reaction.
[a] Levels are influenced by anticoagulation; testing for multiple abnormalities is advisable, because several patients with BCS and portal vein thrombosis had one or more overlapping prothrombotic risk factors.

PORTAL VEIN THROMBOSIS

Extrahepatic obstruction of the portal vein can be caused by thrombosis or by compression or occlusion of the portal trunk or one of its branches by tumors, particularly hepatocellular carcinoma.[1,3,41] In autopsy studies, PVT was found in approximately 1% of the cases, most of them related to cirrhosis or liver cancer with less than one third of the cases attributable to noncirrhotic, nonmalignant PVT.[42] To better characterize those patients without malignancy, two recent consensus conferences[1,41] have recommended the term EHPVO to encompass not only the subjects with recent PVT, but also those with the chronic form known as portal cavernoma. The panel also suggested the categorization as distinct subgroups the cases of intrahepatic PVT and PVT in association with cirrhosis. The following sections address several types of EHPVO beginning with that observed in childhood and concluding with cirrhosis-associated forms of this disorder.

Extrahepatic Portal Vein Obstruction in Childhood

The frequency of EHPVO is higher in Asia and South America, where it affects mainly children. Most of the cases of EHPVO in childhood are either idiopathic[41,43,44] or associated with a past history of umbilical sepsis or umbilical vein catheterization.[45] Even though inherited or acquired thrombophilia were reported to be rare in children with EHPVO,[41,43,44] one Egyptian study has described the association of one or more inherited prothrombotic disorders in up to 63% of the children with EHPVO.[46]

Clinical manifestations in children are mainly a result of portal hypertension.[41,47,48] Most have chronic EHPVO with portal cavernoma disclosed by ultrasound (US) or by MRI or CT angiogram. Variceal bleeding is the most common presentation, but cholestasis caused by portal biliopathy (biliary abnormalities including strictures as a result of extrinsic bile duct compression by dilated venous collaterals), growth retardation, and abdominal distension as a result of splenomegaly or pancytopenia caused by hypersplenism may also occur at presentation. The natural history of EHPVO is usually benign. However, some patients may develop signs of liver failure, which may be ascribed to concurrent hepatitis B or C or liver dysfunction as a result of parenchymal extinction.[49] Management of EHPVO in children is based on uncontrolled studies and includes sclerotherapy or endoscopic band ligation (EBL) for the control of acute variceal bleeding and EBL and/or beta-blockers for secondary prophylaxis.

Anticoagulation should be restricted to those subjects with recognizable prothrombotic disorders. Portal biliopathy treatment is advised only for symptomatic cases, preferably by endoscopic therapy.[41] Surgical shunts, particularly distal splenorenal shunts, have been performed for variceal bleeding or portal biliopathy refractory to endoscopic therapy, but the use of mesenteric to left portal vein bypass (Rex shunt) has been advocated to be more physiologic, as it restores portal venous blood flow to the liver via the left portal vein in the Rex recessus.[50,51] The use of Rex shunts has been associated with excellent long-term outcomes including no further bleeding episodes from varices, partial or complete regression of splenomegaly, improvement in platelet and leukocyte counts, and normalization of coagulation abnormalities in most of the surgically treated subjects.[39] These findings altogether have led some authorities to consider this surgical procedure as the therapy of choice for symptomatic EHPVO in children, when technically feasible.[51]

Nonmalignant, Noncirrhotic Extrahepatic Portal Vein Obstruction in Adults

Nontumoral EHPVO in adults can be classified according to presentation as acute PVT or chronic EHPVO, as well as to the presence or absence of cirrhosis, which is discussed separately in the next section.[3] Portal vein thrombosis can also occur in association with other liver diseases caused by prothrombotic disorders such as BCS or noncirrhotic portal hypertension (NCPH).[52] In adults, noncirrhotic, nontumoral EHPVO is quite rare and accounts for less than 10% of the cases of portal hypertension with fewer than 400 patients reported from three reference centers in Europe.[3,8,9,53]

Clinical findings and management options vary according to the type of EHPVO. Acute or recent PVT is characterized by recent occlusion of the portal vein by a thrombus that can be associated or not with symptoms of abdominal pain and diarrhea, as well as signs of systemic inflammatory response or sepsis in case of pylephlebitis.[3] Severity depends on the extent of involvement of the portal venous system. Bloody diarrhea, ascitis, and ileus are more common in severe superior mesenteric vein involvement that may lead to mesenteric ischemia with bowel perforation and septic shock. The diagnosis is usually performed by US, which shows hyperechoic material in the portal vein with downstream dilatation of the portal venous system with no flow detected by Doppler imaging (**Fig. 1**).

Chronic EHPVO is the late-stage sequela of PVT usually defined by the presence of portal cavernoma, characterized by replacement of the portal vein by fibrous tissue and development of periportal collateral vessels bypassing the obstructed portal vein segment.[3,41] Chronic EHPVO leads to portal hypertension with a higher frequency of bleeding from ectopic varices when compared with cirrhosis.[41] Other less frequent manifestations of chronic EHPVO include portal cholangiopathy and hepatic encephalopathy.[3,41,54] Portal cholangiopathy is caused by encasement of bile ducts by dilated peribiliar collaterals leading to irregularities and strictures of the biliary tree particularly at the hilum. These abnormalities may be similar to those observed in

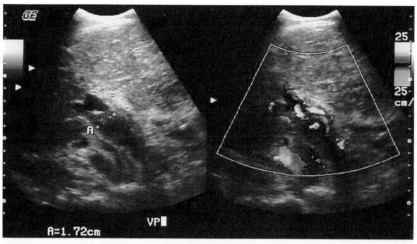

Fig. 1. Doppler ultrasound showing echogenic material in the portal vein with downstream dilatation of the portal venous system and no flow detected by Doppler imaging. (*Courtesy of* Magid Abud, MD, Salvador, Bahia, Brazil.)

primary sclerosing cholangitis and have been reported in up to 80% to 100% of the patients adequately examined by endoscopic retrograde cholangiopancreatography (ERCP) or by magnetic resonance cholangiopancreatography (MRCP). Signs and symptoms of cholestasis or cholangitis are nevertheless quite uncommon. Overt hepatic encephalopathy is rare and is due to the presence of large shunts, but minimal hepatic encephalopathy has been reported in 50% of the patients with chronic EHPVO when assessed by neuropsychological tests, brain MRI imaging, or the oral glutamine challenge test.[54] Diagnosis of chronic EHPVO is usually made by imaging with US and MRI or CT (**Fig. 2**).

The natural history of acute and chronic EHPVO in adults is often relatively benign. Survival is frequently more related to the presence or absence of an associated disorder. In the absence of cirrhosis, massive superior mesenteric vein thrombosis, and cancer, a survival rate of 81% at 10 years has been reported.[53] Mortality is usually related to associated clinical disorders, recurrent thrombotic events, or to the occurrence of massive variceal bleeding.

Because of their rarity, most of the management options and treatment strategies for acute and chronic EHPVO are not based on strong scientific evidence. Guidelines endorsed by the Asian Pacific Association for the Study of the Liver and the Baveno IV Consensus Workshop have been recently published addressing recommendations regarding the current knowledge on acute and chronic EHPVO.[1,41] Management of acute or recent PVT includes treatment of associated infectious or inflammatory disorders and therapy directed toward recanalization of the portal vein, prevention of thrombus extension into the superior mesenteric veins, as well as recurrent thrombosis in those subjects with recognizable prothrombotic risk factors. Based on retrospective analysis of selected cohorts of patients,[55,56] anticoagulation has been recommended in acute PVT for at least 3 months, with the suggestion that it may be lifelong in those subjects with prothrombotic disorders.[1,41] This strategy has been associated with high rates of recanalization of the portal vein with few bleeding events and no mortality as well as no progression to cavernoma and portal hypertension attributable to chronic EHPVO. Recently, one multicentric prospective study

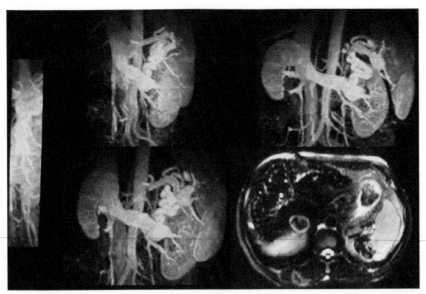

Fig. 2. MR angiography in a patient with cavernous transformation of portal vein. Esophageal varices (on the left): no delineation of the portal vein, enlargement of the splenic vein, and left renal vein because of the presence of a large spontaneous splenorenal shunt. (*Courtesy of* Helio Braga, MD, Salvador, Bahia, Brazil.)

involving 105 patients has shown a recanalization rate of 44% at 1 year after anticoagulation, which was higher in subjects with recent PVT without ascitis. No recurrence of splanchnic vein thrombosis was reported and mortality was 2%.[57]

Several surgical and interventional procedures, including mechanical thrombectomy, systemic or percutaneous transcatheter thrombolysis, angioplasty, or transjugular intrahepatic portosystemic shunt (TIPS), have been performed in subjects with PVT.[58,59] These techniques were shown to be feasible when performed at referral centers and efficacious in selected patients, but major adverse events have been reported in up to 60% of the patients treated by interventional radiology.[58] The Asian consensus has considered percutaneous transhepatic permeation of the portal vein only in patients with progressive recent EHPVO with signs of ongoing mesenteric ischemia despite anticoagulation.[41]

There are no evidence-based data regarding the role of anticoagulation for chronic EHPVO; however, both consensus documents recommend it for patients with known prothrombotic disorders because of the risk of thrombosis recurrence. One retrospective study from France reported long-term results of anticoagulation for 84 subjects with chronic EHPVO. Bleeding events were related to large varices at admission and severity of bleeding was similar in patients with and without anticoagulation. Thrombotic events were related to the presence of thrombophilia or absence of anticoagulation. Mortality was 7% and was not related to anticoagulation.[56] Management of portal hypertension in subjects with chronic EHPVO is less clear when compared with cirrhotic patients because of the lack of controlled data. There is no consensus regarding the best strategy for primary prophylaxis of variceal bleeding. Regarding the control of acute bleeding episodes, endoscopic therapy is recommended with no data on the use of pharmacologic therapy. For secondary prophylaxis, endoscopic therapy is effective, but there are no data on beta-blockers.[1,41] Portal biliopathy with dominant strictures should be treated when symptomatic with therapeutic endoscopy. Shunt surgery is advised in case of endoscopic failure.[1,41]

Portal Vein Thrombosis in Chronic Liver Disease

The prevalence of EHPVO in cirrhosis is estimated at 1%, increasing in accordance with disease progression to 8% to 15% of the patients with Child B or C CLD.[60,61] Symptoms are observed in half of them, either variceal bleeding or abdominal pain with or without mesenteric ischemia. Apart from advanced liver disease, other risk factors recognized for PVT in cirrhotic patients were male sex, previous treatment for portal hypertension, splenomegaly, and alcoholic liver disease, as well as the presence of inherited prothrombotic disorders, particularly factor II G20210A mutation.[60,62]

The frequency of PVT was also reported to rise in patients on the waiting list for orthotopic liver transplantation (OLT) from 8% at admission to 15% at the time of OLT.[61] In this regard, the occurrence of PVT has been associated with higher incidence of postoperative complications and mortality after OLT, particularly in those subjects with complete occlusion of the portal vein with or without involvement of the superior mesenteric vein.[61,63] Based on these findings, Francoz and colleagues[61] from the Beaujon group have attempted to institute anticoagulation to patients with PVT on the waiting list for OLT. They have described partial or complete recanalization in 42% of the treated subjects with no major adverse event reported.

BUDD–CHIARI SYNDROME

Budd–Chiari syndrome is an uncommon and heterogeneous group of disorders characterized by hepatic venous outflow obstruction at any level from the small hepatic veins to the junction of the IVC and the right atrium.[7,64] By definition, outflow obstruction because of heart failure or veno-occlusive disease secondary to nonthrombotic obstruction of the hepatic microcirculation are not considered as variants of BCS.[7]

The prevalence of BCS is estimated as 1:100,000, with fewer than 300 patients reported from three tertiary referral centers in the Netherlands, France, and the United States.[65,66] Obstruction of the hepatic venous outflow tract is classified according to its anatomic impairment, as at the small hepatic veins, large hepatic veins, or IVC (**Table 4**). Obstruction can occur at more than one of these sites, particularly involving the large hepatic veins and IVC.[7] Obstruction of the IVC is more common in the East and is associated with increased frequency of hepatocellular carcinoma.[2] In the West, it is more often found in subjects with factor V Leiden mutation or Behcet's disease. On the other hand, isolated involvement of small hepatic veins is more commonly observed in subjects with paroxysmal nocturnal hemoglobinuria.[2]

It can also be classified as primary when the obstruction results from an endoluminal thrombus or by thrombosis-associated webs, which are now recognized as late-stage sequelae of thrombosis,[21,61] or as secondary when there is an extrinsic invasion or compression of the hepatic veins or IVC by tumors or non-neoplastic mass-forming lesions such as cysts or abscesses (**Table 5**).[7,67] For practical purposes, BCS is considered as primary when no extrinsic causes of secondary obstruction are found by current imaging techniques. Several other classifications based on clinical disease severity or duration such as acute, subacute, and chronic BCS or fulminant BCS have been proposed based on putative differences in prognosis and management.[68–72] However, these classifications are recommended only for descriptive purposes, as they have not been validated in prospective studies and also have not been endorsed because of the lack of well-established criteria for their definition.[7]

Table 4
Classification of Budd–Chiari syndrome according to site of obstruction

Site of Obstruction	Frequency According to Imaging Techniques	Criteria
Small hepatic veins	NA	Involvement of veins that cannot be clearly shown on hepatic venograms or ultrasound, including terminal hepatic veins, and intercalated and interlobular veins
Large hepatic veins[a]	50%	Involvement of veins that are regularly seen on hepatic venograms and ultrasound, including segmental branches of hepatic veins
Inferior vena cava (IVC)	2%	Involvement of one segment of the IVC, which extends from the entry level of the right, middle, and left hepatic veins to the junction between the IVC and the right atrium
Combined obstruction	47%	Involvement of the large hepatic veins and IVC

Abbreviation: NA, not applicable.

[a] Pure hepatic vein involvement is more frequent in Western when compared with Eastern countries.[65]

Data from Janssen HL, Garcia-Pagan JC, Elias E, et al. Budd–Chiari syndrome: a review by an expert panel. J Hepatol 2003;38:364–71; and Plessier A, Denninger MH, Casadevall N, et al. Relevance of the criteria commonly used to diagnose myeloproliferative disorder in patients with splanchnic vein thrombosis. Br J Haematol 2005;129:553–60.

The clinical course of BCS can vary markedly, ranging from asymptomatic disease to fulminant liver failure,[68–72] depending on the speed of occlusion, the extent of hepatic vein involvement, and on whether a venous collateral circulation has developed to decompress the liver sinusoids. Most patients present painful hepatomegaly and ascites.[70–72] Differential diagnosis with sinusoidal obstruction syndrome (SOS) and cardiac insufficiency is important, as these entities may present with similar clinical features.[7] Heart failure can be ruled out by careful physical examination and echocardiography when appropriate. SOS, formerly known as veno-occlusive disease,[2,73] usually occurs after myeloablative hematopoietic stem cell transplantation, when its diagnosis is usually straightforward. However, when SOS is associated with ingestion of pyrrolizidine alkaloids or other drugs, liver biopsy is usually required for its diagnosis.

Table 5
Classification of Budd–Chiari syndrome according to etiology

Etiology	Criteria
Primary	Hepatic venous outflow obstruction resulting from endoluminal venous lesion (thrombosis, webs, endophlebitis). Of note, webs are now recognized as late-stage sequel of thrombosis.
Secondary	Hepatic venous outflow obstruction caused by invasion or obstruction from a lesion outside the hepatic outflow venous system (tumor, abscess, cysts).

Adapted from Janssen HL, Garcia-Pagan JC, Elias E, et al. Budd–Chiari syndrome: a review by an expert panel. J Hepatol 2003;38:364–71; with permission.

According to recommendations from an expert panel report,[7] BCS should be suspected in patients with abrupt onset of ascites and painful hepatomegaly, massive ascites without major impairment in liver function, fulminant hepatic failure associated with hepatomegaly and ascites, or liver disease associated with inherited or acquired thrombophilia, as well as in subjects with unexplained chronic liver disease. Ascites fluid analysis, which typically shows high protein, high albumin gradient in the absence of heart failure can also be a practical clue to the presence of BCS. The diagnosis is usually established by Doppler ultrasonography (DU), which demonstrates thrombosis or absence of hepatic veins; absent, reversed, or turbulent flow; or occurrence of collateral hepatic venous circulation, as well as enlargement of the caudate lobe. Sensitivity and specificity for DU ranges from 75% to 85%.[72,74] Nonvisualized or tortuous hepatic veins are common but nonspecific sonographic findings of BCS, while intrahepatic or subcapsular venous collaterals are sensitive sonographic findings (**Fig. 3**).[72,74–76] CT is superior to DU to assess IVC involvement and to reveal liver perfusion defects (**Fig. 4**).[74]

MRI has been recommended as the second method of investigation (**Fig. 5**),[7] as it allows better delineation of the vascular anatomy of splanchnic vessels without use of contrast agents and is also able to better differentiate acute from chronic BCS.[67,76] Venography is usually performed when noninvasive imaging techniques fail to provide clear-cut diagnosis of BCS in patients with a high index of suspicion of the disease or when surgical shunts are a treatment option to assess the occurrence of IVC

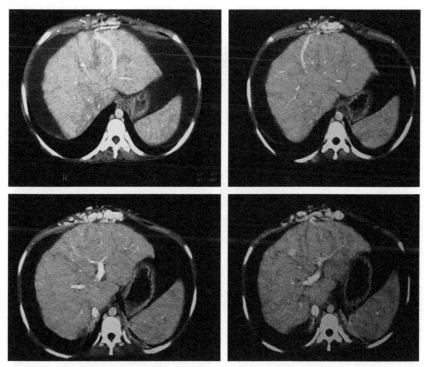

Fig. 3. CT demonstrates absence of hepatic veins, enlargement of the caudate lobe, and the presence of intrahepatic and subcapsular venous collaterals. (*Courtesy of* Luciana Costa Silva, MD, PhD, Minas Gerais, Brazil.)

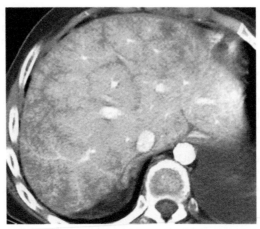

Fig. 4. CT scanning showing diffuse perfusion defects and absence of the hepatic veins.

obstruction by pressure measurements. Liver biopsy is rarely used for diagnostic purposes but it has been recently used for prognosis.[77] In this regard, the presence of acute injuries associated with chronic lesions on liver biopsy has been associated with shortened survival.[77]

Prognosis has been improved markedly in recent years, with survival rates of 77% to 82%, 65% to 69%, and 57% to 62%, at 1, 5, and 10 years, respectively,[65,78,79] probably because of improved recognition of BCS, particularly asymptomatic cases, and more frequent use of anticoagulation.[2,78] The risk of death is highest within the

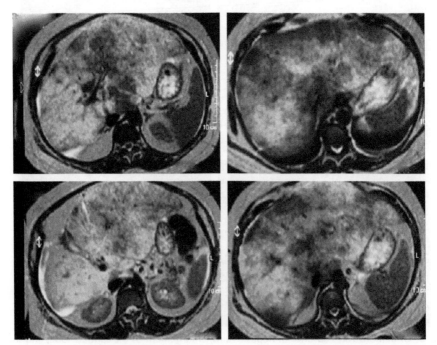

Fig. 5. MRI in a patient with absence of the hepatic veins. (*Courtesy of* Luciana Costa Silva, MD, PhD, Minas Gerais, Brazil.)

first 1 to 2 years after diagnosis, whereas patients surviving beyond 2 years have excellent long-term survival rates.[37–39] Adverse outcomes have been associated with age at presentation, poor response of ascites to diuretics, Child-Pugh score, and renal failure,[78] as well as the occurrence of encephalopathy, ascitis, enlarged prothrombin time, and hyperbilirrubinemia.[65]

Strategies for the treatment of BCS are not evidence-based because of the rarity of this disorder and the lack of randomized controlled trials evaluating current available treatment options, including medical management aimed at control of underlying diseases and complications of portal hypertension, as well as anticoagulation and surgical treatment with portosystemic shunts (PSS) or OLT and interventional radiology with angioplasty coupled or not with thrombolysis and TIPS.[80] Two expert opinion reports have been published regarding the management of BCS.[1,7]

Management of ascites and prevention and treatment of portal hypertensive bleeding in patients with BCS are not different when compared with cirrhotic patients and subjects with EHPVO,[1] but data concerning treatment issues in BCS are scanty even when compared with EHPVO. Anticoagulation is recommended in the presence of recent or long-standing thrombosis to allow recanalization or to avoid thrombus progression or recurrence. Surgical or radiological approaches to relieve sinusoidal pressure in patients with BCS have been advocated,[80] but they were not associated with improvement in survival[65,78] and are now considered appropriate only for symptomatic patients who do not improve with medical management.[1,2,7] Interventional radiology using percutaneous thrombolysis and angioplasty with or without stenting could be a first-line strategy for selected patients with recent thrombosis or subjects with short-length stenosis of the IVC or hepatic veins with excellent outcomes reported from centers with skillful radiology teams.[19,81]

Use of PSS was advocated as a definite measure to relieve sinusoidal hypertension with the potential to reverse hepatic necrosis and prevent cirrhosis. It is now largely replaced by TIPS. However, both treatment modalities have been associated with high rates of shunt dysfunction, requiring revision and leading to increased morbidity.[2,81,82] Liver transplantation is required when the aforementioned treatment strategies fail in patients with a progressive downhill course with 1-, 5-, and 10-year survival rates of 76%, 71%, and 68%, respectively.[82] Renal failure and presence of PSS and/or TIPS before OLT were associated with shortened survival. Anticoagulation is required after OLT to prevent recurrence of thrombosis, which may occur in 2% to 27% of the cases.[82,83]

ASSOCIATION OF BUDD–CHIARI SYNDROME, EXTRAHEPATIC PORTAL VEIN OBSTRUCTION, AND NONCIRRHOTIC PORTAL HYPERTENSION

Extrahepatic portal vein obstruction may overlap with other vascular disorders of the liver, particularly with BCS and NCPH. In a multicenter European cohort of BCS, EHPVO was observed in 18% of the affected subjects.[52] The clinical presentation was similar irrespective of the presence of EHPVO, however two or more prothrombotic risk factors tended to be more frequent in patients with associated splanchnic vein thrombosis. Survival also tended to be reduced in subjects with BCS-associated EHPVO. Hepatoportal sclerosis is another vascular disorder of the liver that is frequent in the East and leads to NCPH.[41,84] Thrombosis of the medium to small portal veins has been recently linked to its pathogenesis.[41] In a retrospective review of 28 Western patients followed for 7.6 years, EHPVO was shown to develop in 46% of the cases.[85] Most of those subjects had associated prothrombotic disorders, particularly chronic MPD.

SUMMARY

Nonmalignant, noncirrhotic EHPVO and Budd–Chiari syndrome are mainly caused by several heterogeneous inherited and acquired prothrombotic disorders. Investigation of thrombophilia can be difficult in this setting and a formal hematological consultation is usually required. Variceal bleeding caused by portal hypertension is the most frequent clinical manifestation of EHPVO, but cholestasis caused by portal biliopathy, growth retardation, splenomegaly, and pancytopenia caused by hypersplenism and hepatic encephalopathy may also occur. Treatment options are based on uncontrolled data and include anticoagulation to prevent thrombosis extension or recurrence and prophylaxis as well as treatment of complications of portal hypertension. In children, excellent long-term outcomes have been reported with the use of mesenteric to left portal vein bypass (Rex shunt). The natural history of nonmalignant, noncirrhotic EHPVO in adults is relatively benign and survival is directly related to the presence of an associated prothrombotic disorder.

The clinical course of BCS can vary from asymptomatic disease to fulminant liver failure, depending on the speed and the extent of the occlusion. Most patients present with painful hepatomegaly and high-protein fluid ascites. Doppler ultrasonography is usually required for diagnosis. Prognosis has improved markedly in recent years, but age at presentation; poor response of ascitis to diuretics; Child-Pugh score; and the occurrence of renal failure, hepatic encephalopathy, increased prothrombin time, and hyperbilirrubinemia have been associated with adverse outcomes. Strategies for the treatment of BCS are not evidence-based and should be individualized. Medical management includes anticoagulation for those subjects with prothrombotic risk factors and control of the complications of portal hypertension, such as ascitis and variceal bleeding. Other treatment options include surgical portosystemic shunts, TIPS, or liver transplantation. Recently, medical management has been favored as first-line therapy, because surgical and radiological approaches to relieve sinusoidal pressure in patients with BCS have not been shown to improve survival. In patients with failure of medical therapy and a progressive downhill course, TIPS and liver transplantation are advocated with excellent long-term survival.

REFERENCES

1. De Franchis R. Evolving consensus in portal hypertension. Report of the Baveno IV consensus workshop on methodology of diagnosis and therapy in portal hypertension. J Hepatol 2005;43:167–76.
2. Valla DC. The diagnosis and management of the Budd–Chiari syndrome: consensus and controversies. Hepatology 2003;38:793–803.
3. Condat B, Valla D. Nonmalignant portal vein thrombosis in adults. Nat Clin Pract Gastroenterol Hepatol 2006;3:505–15.
4. Middeldorp S, Levi M. Thrombophilia: an update. Semin Thromb Hemost 2007; 33:563–72.
5. Simioni P, Tormene D, Spiezia L, et al. Inherited thrombophilia and venous thromboembolism. Semin Thromb Hemost 2006;32:700–8.
6. Franco RF, Trip MP, Reitsma PH. Genetic variations of the hemostatic system as a risk factor for venous and arterial thrombotic disease. Curr Genomics 2003;4: 1–21.
7. Janssen HL, Garcia-Pagan JC, Elias E, et al. Budd–Chiari syndrome: a review by an expert panel. J Hepatol 2003;38:364–71.
8. Primignani M, Martinelli I, Bucciarelli P, et al. Risk factors for thrombophilia in extrahepatic portal vein obstruction. Hepatology 2005;41:603–8.

9. Denninger MH, Chait Y, Casadevall N, et al. Cause of portal or hepatic venous thrombosis in adults: the role of multiple concurrent factors. Hepatology 2000; 31:587–91.
10. Janssen HL, Meinardi JR, Vleggaar FP, et al. Factor V Leiden mutation, prothrombin gene mutation, and deficiencies in coagulation inhibitors associated with Budd–Chiari syndrome and portal vein thrombosis: results of a case-control study. Blood 2000;96:2364–8.
11. Bhattacharyya M, Makharia G, Kannan M, et al. Inherited prothrombotic defects in Budd–Chiari syndrome and portal vein thrombosis: a study from North India. Am J Clin Pathol 2004;121:844–7.
12. Mohanty D, Shetty S, Ghosh K, et al. Hereditary thrombophilia as a cause of Budd–Chiari syndrome: a study from western India. Hepatology 2001;34:666–70.
13. Brie JB. Budd–Chiari syndrome and portal vein thrombosis associated with myeloproliferative disorders: diagnosis and management. Semin Thromb Hemost 2006;32:208–18.
14. Deltenre P, Denninger MH, Hillaire S, et al. Factor V Leiden related Budd–Chiari syndrome. Gut 2001;48:264–8.
15. Aydinli M, Bayraktar Y. Budd–Chiari syndrome: etiology, pathogenesis and diagnosis. World J Gastroenterol 2007;13:2693–6.
16. Li XM, Wei YF, Hao HL, et al. Hyperhomocysteinemia and the MTHFR C677T mutation in Budd–Chiari syndrome. Am J Hematol 2002;71:11–4.
17. Lim W, Crowther MA. Antiphospholipid antibodies: a critical review of the literature. Curr Opin Hematol 2007;14:494–9.
18. Cohn DM, Roshani S, Middeldorp S. Thrombophilia and venous thromboembolism: implications for testing. Semin Thromb Hemost 2007;33:573–81.
19. Sharma S, Kumar SI, Poddar U, et al. Factor V Leiden and prothrombin gene G20210A mutations are uncommon in portal vein thrombosis in India. Indian J Gastroenterol 2006;25:236–9.
20. Valla DC. Portal vein thrombosis and prothrombotic disorders. J Gastroenterol Hepatol 1999;14:1051–2.
21. Valla DC. Hepatic venous outflow tract obstruction etiopathogenesis: Asia versus the West. J Gastroenterol Hepatol 2004;19:S204–11.
22. Heit JA. Thrombophilia: common questions on laboratory assessment and management. Educational Book. Hematology 2007;127–35.
23. Chait Y, Condat B, Cazals-Hatem D, et al. Relevance of the criteria commonly used to diagnose myeloproliferative disorder in patients with splanchnic vein thrombosis. Br J Haematol 2005;129:553–60.
24. Patel RK, Nicholas CL, Heneghan MA, et al. Prevalence of the activating *JAK2* tyrosine kinase mutation V617F in the Budd–Chiari syndrome. Gastroenterology 2006;130:2031–8.
25. Thurmes PJ, Steensma DP. Elevated serum erythropoietin levels in patients with Budd–Chiari syndrome secondary to polycythemia vera: clinical implications for the role of JAK2 mutation analysis. Eur J Haematol 2006;77:57–60.
26. Colaizzo D, Amitrano L, Tiscia GL, et al. The JAK2 V617F mutation frequently occurs in patients with portal and mesenteric venous thrombosis. J Thromb Haemost 2007;5:55–61.
27. Jones AV, Kreil S, Zoi K, et al. Widespread occurrence of the *JAK2* V617F mutation in chronic myeloproliferative disorders. Blood 2005;106:2162–8.
28. De Stefano V, Fiorini A, Rossi E, et al. Incidence of the JAK2 V617F mutation among patients with splanchnic or cerebral venous thrombosis and without overt chronic myeloproliferative disorders. J Thromb Haemost 2007;5:708–14.

29. Kaushansky K. On the molecular origins of the chronic myeloproliferative disorders: it all makes sense. Blood 2005;105:4258–63.

30. Dudley JM, Westwood N, Leonard S, et al. Primary polycythemia: positive diagnosis using the differential response of primitive and mature erythroid progenitors to erythropoietin, interleukin 3 and alpha-interferon. Br J Haematol 1990;75:188–94.

31. Dainiak N, Hoffman R, Lebowitz AI, et al. Erythropoietin-dependent primary pure erythrocytosis. Blood 1979;53:1076–84.

32. Eridani S, Dudley JM, Sawyer BM, et al. Erythropoietic colonies in a serum-free system: results in primary proliferative polycythemia and thrombocythemias. Br J Haematol 1987;67:387–91.

33. Levine RL, Wernig G. Role of JAK-STAT signaling in the pathogenesis of myeloproliferative disorders. Hematology Am Soc Hematol Educ Program 2006;510: 233–9.

34. Kralovics R, Passamonti F, Buser AS, et al. A gain-of-function mutation of JAK2 in myeloproliferative disorders. N Engl J Med 2005;352:1779–90.

35. Kiladjian JJ, Cervantes F, Leebeek FW, et al. The impact of JAK2 and MPL mutations on diagnosis and prognosis of splanchnic vein thrombosis: a report on 241 cases. Blood 2008;111:4922–9.

36. Murad SD, Plessier A, Hernandez Guerra M, et al. A prospective follow-up study on 163 patients with Budd–Chiari syndrome: results from the European network for vascular disorders of the liver (EM_VIE). J Hepatol 2007;46:S4 [abstract].

37. Levine JS, Branch DW, Rauch J. The antiphospholipid syndrome. N Engl J Med 2002;346:752–63.

38. Miyakis S, Lockshin MD, Atsumi T, et al. International consensus statement on an update of the classification criteria for definite antiphospholipid syndrome (APS). J Thromb Haemost 2006;4:296–306.

39. Superina R, Bambini DA, Lokar J, et al. Correction of extrahepatic portal vein thrombosis by the mesenteric to left portal vein bypass. Ann Surg 2006;243: 515–21.

40. Ziakas PD, Poulou LS, Rokas GI, et al. Thrombosis in paroxysmal nocturnal hemoglobinuria: sites, risks, outcome. An overview. J Thromb Haemost 2007;5: 642–5.

41. Sarin SK, Sollano JD, Chawla YK, et al. Consensus on extra-hepatic portal vein obstruction. Liver Int 2006;26:512–9.

42. Ogren M, Bergqvist D, Bjorck M, et al. Portal vein thrombosis: prevalence, patient characteristics and lifetime risk: a population study based on 23,796 consecutive autopsies. World J Gastroenterol 2006;12:2115–9.

43. Pinto RB, Silveira TR, Bandinelli E, et al. Portal vein thrombosis in children and adolescents: the low prevalence of hereditary thrombophilic disorders. J Pediatr Surg 2004;39:1356–61.

44. Pugliese RPS, Porta G, D'Amico EA, et al. Risk factors in children and adolescents with portal vein thrombosis (PVT) and portal hypertension. Hepatology 1998;28:551A.

45. Alvarez F. Risk of portal obstruction in newborns. J Pediatr 2006;148:715–6.

46. El-Karaksy H, El-Koofy N, El-Hawary M, et al. Prevalence of factor V Leiden mutation and other hereditary thrombophilic factors in Egyptian children with portal vein thrombosis: results of a single-center case-control study. Ann Hematol 2004;83:712–5.

47. Lykavieris P, Gauthier F, Hadchouel P, et al. Risk of gastrointestinal bleeding during adolescence and early adulthood in children with portal vein obstruction. J Pediatr 2000;136:805–8.

48. Alvarez F, Bernard O, Brunelle F, et al. Portal obstruction in children. I. Clinical investigation and hemorrhage risk. J Pediat 1983;103:696–702.
49. Rangari M, Gupta R, Jain M, et al. Hepatic dysfunction in patients with extrahepatic portal venous obstruction. Liver Int 2003;23:434–9.
50. De Ville de Goyet J, Gibbs P, Clapuyt P, et al. Original extrahilar approach for hepatic portal revascularization and relief of extrahepatic portal hypertension related to later portal vein thrombosis after pediatric liver transplantation. Long-term results. Transplantation 1996;62:71–5.
51. Superina R, Shneider B, Emre S, et al. Surgical guidelines for the management of extra-hepatic portal vein obstruction. Pediatr Transplant 2006;10:908–13.
52. Murad SD, Valla DC, de Groen PC, et al. Pathogenesis and treatment of Budd–Chiari syndrome combined with portal vein thrombosis. Am J Gastroenterol 2006;101:83–90.
53. Janssen HL, Wijnhourd A, Haagsma EB, et al. Extrahepatic portal vein thrombosis: aetiology and determinants of survival. Gut 2001;49:720–4.
54. Mínguez B, García-Pagán JC, Bosch J, et al. Noncirrhotic portal vein thrombosis exhibits neuropsychological and MR changes consistent with minimal hepatic encephalopathy. Hepatology 2006;43:707–14.
55. Condat B, Pessione F, Hillaire S, et al. Recent portal or mesenteric venous thrombosis: increased recognition and frequent recanalization on anticoagulant therapy. Hepatology 2000;32:466–70.
56. Condat B, Pessione F, Hillaire S, et al. Current outcome of portal vein thrombosis in adults: risk and benefit of anticoagulant therapy. Gastroenterology 2001;120:490–7.
57. Plessier A, Murad SD, Hernandez Guerra M, et al. A prospective multicentric follow-up study on 105 patients with acute portal vein thrombosis (PVT): results from the European network for vascular disorders of the liver (EM-VIE). Hepatology 2007;46:309A [abstract].
58. Hollingshead M, Burke CT, Mauro MA, et al. Transcatheter thrombolytic therapy for acute mesenteric and portal vein thrombosis. J Vasc Interv Radiol 2005;16:651–61.
59. Senzolo M, Tibbals J, Cholongitas E, et al. Transjugular intrahepatic portosystemic shunt for portal vein thrombosis with and without cavernous transformation. Aliment Pharmacol Ther 2006;23:767–75.
60. Amitrano L, Guardascione MA, Brancaccio V, et al. Risk factors and clinical presentation of portal vein thrombosis in patients with liver cirrhosis. J Hepatol 2004;40:736–41.
61. Francoz C, Belghiti J, Vilgrain V, et al. Splanchnic vein thrombosis in candidates for liver transplantation: usefulness of screening and anticoagulation. Gut 2006;54:691–7.
62. Amitrano L, Brancaccio V, Guardascione MA, et al. Inherited coagulation disorders in cirrhotic patients with portal vein thrombosis. Hepatology 2000;31:345–8.
63. Yerdel MA, Gunson B, Mirza D, et al. Portal vein thrombosis in adults undergoing liver transplantation: risk factors, screening, management, and outcome. Transplantation 2000;69:1873–81.
64. Ludwig J, Hashimoto E, McGill DB, et al. Classification of hepatic venous outflow obstruction: ambiguous terminology of the Budd–Chiari syndrome. Mayo Clin Proc 1990;65:51–5.
65. Murad SD, Valla DC, de Groen PC, et al. Determinants of survival and the effect of portosystemic shunting in patients with Budd–Chiari syndrome. Hepatology 2004;39:500–8.

66. Okuda K. Membranous obstruction of the inferior vena cava (obliterative hepato-cavopathy, Okuda). J Gastroenterol Hepatol 2001;16:1179–83.
67. Zimmerman MA, Cameron AM, Ghobrial RM. Budd–Chiari syndrome. Clin Liver Dis 2006;10:259–73.
68. Menon KVN, Shah V, Kamath PS. Current concepts: the Budd–Chiari Syndrome. N Engl J Med 2004;350:578–85.
69. Hadengue A, Poliquin M, Vilgrain V, et al. The changing scene of hepatic vein thrombosis: recognition of asymptomatic cases. Gastroenterology 1994;106: 1042–7.
70. Dilawari JB, Bambery P, Chawla Y, et al. Hepatic outflow obstruction (Budd–Chiari syndrome). Experience with 177 patients and a review of the literature. Medicine (Baltimore) 1994;73:21–36.
71. Mahmoud AE, Mendoza A, Meshikhes AN, et al. Clinical spectrum, investigations and treatment of Budd–Chiari syndrome. Q J Med 1996;89:37–43.
72. Bolondi L, Gaiani S, Li Bassi S, et al. Diagnosis of Budd–Chiari syndrome by pulsed Doppler ultrasound. Gastroenterology 1991;100:1324–31.
73. DeLeve LD, Shulman HM, McDonald GB. Toxic injury to hepatic sinusoids: sinu-soidal obstruction syndrome (veno-occlusive disease). Semin Liver Dis 2002;22: 27–42.
74. Kamath P. Budd–Chiari syndrome: radiologic findings. Liver Transp 2006;12: S21–2.
75. Chawla Y, Kumar S, Dhiman RK, et al. Duplex Doppler sonography in patients with Budd–Chiari syndrome. J Gastroenterol Hepatol 1999;14:904–7.
76. Brancatelli G, Vilgrain V, Federle MP, et al. Budd–Chiari syndrome: spectrum of imaging findings. AJR Am J Roentgenol 2007;188(2):168–76.
77. Langlet P, Escolano S, Valla D, et al. Clinicopathological forms and prognostic index in Budd–Chiari syndrome. J Hepatol 2003;39:496–501.
78. Zeitoun G, Escolano S, Hadengue A, et al. Outcome of Budd–Chiari syndrome: a multivariate analysis of factors related to survival including surgical portosyste-mic shunting. Hepatology 1999;30:84–9.
79. Orloff MJ, Daily PO, Orloff SL, et al. A 27-year experience with surgical treatment of Budd–Chiari syndrome. Ann Surg 2000;232:340–52.
80. Klein AS. Management of Budd–Chiari syndrome. Liver Transpl 2006;12:S23–8.
81. Eapen CE, Velissaris D, Heydtmann M, et al. Favourable medium term outcome following hepatic vein recanalisation and/or transjugular intrahepatic portosyste-mic shunt for Budd Chiari syndrome. Gut 2006;55:878–84.
82. Mentha G, Giostra E, Majno PE, et al. Liver transplantation for Budd-Chiari syndrome: a European study on 248 patients from 51 centres. J Hepatol 2006; 44:520–8.
83. Cruz E, Ascher NL, Roberts JP, et al. High incidence of recurrence and hemato-logic events following liver transplantation for Budd-Chiari syndrome. Clin Trans-plant 2005;19:501–6.
84. Sarin SK, Kumar A. Non-cirrhotic portal hypertension. Clin Liver Dis 2006;10: 627–51.
85. Hillaire S, Bonte E, Denninger M-H, et al. Idiopathic non-cirrhotic intrahepatic portal hypertension in the west: a re-evaluation in 28 patients. Gut 2002;51: 275–80.

Systemic Mastocytosis

Tracy I. George, MD[a],*, Hans-Peter Horny, MD[b]

KEYWORDS

- Systemic mastocytosis • Mast cell • KIT D816V
- Mast cell leukemia

OVERVIEW

Mast cell disease, or mastocytosis, includes a variety of disorders that are characterized by clonal, neoplastic proliferations of mast cells in one or multiple organs, ranging from indolent and isolated proliferations to aggressive and systemic disorders.[1] Mastocytosis is now included in the myeloproliferative neoplasms category in the 2008 World Health Organization (WHO) classification in recognition of the common theme of abnormal protein tyrosine kinase function that characterizes the myeloproliferative neoplasms. The hallmark of most mastocytosis cases is the Asp816Val (D816 V) somatic mutation in the catalytic domain of the *KIT* gene, resulting in enhanced mast cell survival and proliferation owing to constitutive activation of the *KIT* tyrosine kinase activity.[2] The WHO classification of mastocytosis is as follows:

- Cutaneous mastocytosis
- Indolent systemic mastocytosis
- Systemic mastocytosis with associated clonal hematological non–mast cell lineage disease (SM-AHNMD)
- Aggressive systemic mastocytosis
- Mast cell leukemia
- Mast cell sarcoma
- Extracutaneous mastocytoma.

Clinical manifestations are caused by the release of chemical mediators and by infiltration of tissues by neoplastic mast cells. Morphologic detection and immunophenotypic confirmation of mast cells in tissue sections is essential for the diagnosis of mastocytosis. Mast cells can vary from collections of round cells with many fine

---

A version of this article originally appeared in *Surgical Pathology Clinics*, 3:4.

Disclosures: Drs George and Horny are on the Steering Committee for Study CPKC412D2201 for Novartis and are paid consultants.

[a] Department of Pathology, Stanford University School of Medicine, Stanford University Medical Center, 300 Pasteur Drive, Room H1501B, Stanford, CA 94305-5627, USA

[b] Institut für Pathologie, Klinikum Ansbach, Escherichstrasse 6 DE-91522, Ansbach, Germany

* Corresponding author.

E-mail address: tigeorge@stanford.edu

Hematol Oncol Clin N Am 25 (2011) 1067–1083

doi:10.1016/j.hoc.2011.09.012

0889-8588/11/$ – see front matter © 2011 Elsevier Inc. All rights reserved.

basophilic granules to spindled forms with associated fibrosis to blastlike cells with large metachromatic granules, with the latter atypical forms correlating with the more aggressive clinical syndromes. The subtle nature of some mast cell infiltrates can be easily overlooked or masked by accompanying eosinophils, small lymphocytes, and plasma cells.

Classification of mastocytosis into systemic mastocytosis (SM) subtypes requires correlation with clinical and laboratory findings. The WHO classification of mastocytosis separates cutaneous from systemic forms and provides criteria to further subclassify the systemic forms of mastocytosis, based on the presence of specific clinical, laboratory, and pathologic findings (that are divided into "B" and "C" groups) **(Tables 1 and 2).**[2]

Clinical Features

Mastocytosis is clinically heterogeneous, ranging from skin lesions that spontaneously regress to aggressive malignancies with short survival. It can occur at any age with a slight male predominance.[3] In cutaneous mastocytosis, mast cell infiltration is limited to the skin and typically presents in childhood with urticarial symptoms. It has a benign clinical course and may regress spontaneously, often around the time of puberty. In adults, cutaneous disease is more frequently associated with indolent rather than aggressive forms of SM (see the WHO classification listed previously). Thus, in adults presenting with cutaneous disease, careful staging for SM is recommended, including a physical examination, complete blood cell count, total serum tryptase, bone marrow examination, and molecular analysis for the D816 V *KIT* mutation; additional laboratory and radiographic studies may be indicated based on the patient's symptoms and signs of disease. Whereas the bone marrow is almost always involved in SM,[4] the spleen, lymph nodes, liver and gastrointestinal tract, and virtually any organ, can also be affected. Clinical manifestations of SM reflect either mediator release from mast cells or infiltration of mast cells into tissues; they include constitutional signs, skin lesions, mediator-related findings (flushing, syncope, diarrhea, hypotension, headache, and/or abdominal pain), and musculoskeletal disease.

Four major types of SM are known[5]:

1. Indolent systemic mastocytosis
2. Systemic mastocytosis accompanied by an associated hematological non–mast cell disorder (SM-AHNMD)
3. Aggressive systemic mastocytosis and variant lymphadenopathic mastocytosis with eosinophilia
4. Mast cell leukemia.

Table 1
Criteria for systemic mastocytosis[a] Diagnosis requires 1 major and 1 minor criterion or 3 minor criteria

Major	Multifocal dense infiltrates of mast cells in tissue sections[b]
Minor	>25% spindled, immature or atypical mast cells in tissue sections or bone marrow aspirate smears
	Detection of *KIT* D816 V mutation
	Expression of CD2 and/or CD25 in mast cells
	Serum total tryptase persistently exceeds 20 ng/mL[c]

[a] 2008 World Health Organization Diagnostic Criteria for Systemic Mastocytosis.
[b] Infiltrate is ≥15 mast cells in aggregates in bone marrow and/or extracutaneous organs.
[c] Not valid if there is an associated clonal myeloid disorder.

Table 2
"B Findings" and "C Findings" used to subcategorize systemic mastocytosis

B Findings	
1. Increased mast cell burden	>30% mast cell aggregates on bone marrow biopsy and/or total serum tryptase level >200 ng/mL
2. Dysplasia or myeloproliferation	Hypercellular marrow, signs of myelodysplasia or abnormal myeloid proliferation, and normal or slightly abnormal blood counts, without sufficient criteria to diagnose an AHNMD
3. Organomegaly	Palpable hepatomegaly without ascites or signs of liver dysfunction, palpable or radiologic lymphadenopathy (>2 cm), or palpable splenomegaly, without hypersplenism
C Findings	
1. Cytopenias	ANC <1.0 × 10⁹/L; Hb <10 g/dL; or platelets <100 × 10⁹/L
2. Liver	Palpable hepatomegaly with impaired liver function, ascites, and/or portal hypertension
3. Bone	Large osteolytic lesions and/or pathologic fractures
4. Spleen	Palpable splenomegaly with hypersplenism
5. Gastrointestinal	Malabsorption with weight loss and/or hypoalbuminemia

Abbreviations: AHNMD, associated clonal hematologic non–mast cell lineage disease; ANC, absolute neutrophil count; Hb, hemoglobin.

Indolent systemic mastocytosis involves skin and bone marrow and is the most common form of SM. Variants of indolent SM include *bone marrow mastocytosis,* in which no skin disease is present, *smoldering systemic mastocytosis* in which 2 or more "B findings" are present (see **Table 2**), and *well-differentiated (round cell) mastocytosis,* discussed later. Smoldering SM mainly affects older patients and is associated with more constitutional symptoms than the other types of indolent disease.

In *systemic mastocytosis accompanied by an associated hematological non–mast cell disorder* (SM-AHNMD), the associated non–mast cell disorder is usually a myeloid malignancy, but may also include lymphomas or plasma cell neoplasms. Symptoms and prognosis typically reflect the associated non–mast cell disease.

Aggressive systemic mastocytosis is a disorder typically lacking skin lesions and presenting with one or more "C findings" that indicate organ dysfunction owing to mast cell infiltration (see **Table 2**). A variant of aggressive SM is *lymphadenopathic mastocytosis with eosinophilia,* which presents with lymphadenopathy and eosinophilia. This subtype should be differentiated from myeloid/lymphoid neoplasms with *PDGFRA* rearrangements.

The last major type is the rare *mast cell leukemia* (comprising only 1% of SM cases), which also presents without skin lesions and shares the extremely poor prognosis of aggressive SM. Two localized extracutaneous mast cell neoplasms, mast cell sarcoma and extracutaneous mastocytoma, are exceedingly rare and are not discussed in this article.[5]

Microscopic Features

Mast Cell Cytology

The spectrum of reactive and neoplastic mast cell appearances is presented in **Table 3**. Reactive tissue mast cells are small with round, centrally located nuclei,

Table 3
Pathology key features of mast cell proliferations: mast cell morphology

Mast Cell Type	Size/Shape	Nucleus	Nuclear Chromatin	Cytoplasm	Nuclear to Cytoplasmic Ratio	Associated Disorders
Reactive	Small-medium, round or oval	Central, round or oval	Condensed	Well granulated, may be hypo- or degranulated	Low	Reactive mastocytosis
Atypical type I	Elongated cytoplasmic extensions (spindle shaped)	Central or eccentric, oval	Condensed	Hypogranulated, focal granule accumulation without degranulation	Variable	SM, SM-AHNMD
Atypical type II	Variable	Bi- or polylobed	Fine or condensed	Hypogranulated without degranulation	Variable	MCL, MML
Metachromatic[a] blast	Medium-large, round or oval	Prominent nucleoli	Fine	Few metachromatic granules	High	MCL, MML

Abbreviations: ASM, aggressive systemic mastocytosis; BM, bone marrow; MC, mast cell(s); MCL, mast cell leukemia; MML, myelomastocytic leukemia; SM-AHNMD, systemic mastocytosis with an associated clonal hematological non–mast cell lineage disease.

[a] Metachromatic refers to a cell that characteristically takes on a color different from that of the dye with which it is stained; a metachromatic blast has the nuclear features of a blast with many large basophilic cytoplasmic granules.

indistinct to absent nucleoli, and abundant cytoplasm containing faint cytoplasmic granules on hematoxylin and eosin (H&E)-stained tissue sections. In Romanowsky-stained smears, normal mast cells contain tightly packed uniform metachromatic granules with round to oval-shaped nuclei (**Fig. 1**). Neoplastic mast cell morphology has been classified into 3 subtypes (see **Fig. 1**) that are best recognized on bone marrow aspirate smears. The first subtype is the *atypical mast cell type I*, a spindled mast cell with elongated cytoplasmic projections, oval eccentric nuclei, and hypogranulated cytoplasm. The second subtype is the *atypical mast cell type II* or *promastocyte*, with bilobed or polylobed nuclei and typically less cytoplasmic granulation than reactive mast cells. The third subtype is the *metachromatic blast,* which has a high nuclear to cytoplasmic ratio, fine nuclear chromatin, prominent nucleoli, and several metachromatic granules. Atypical type I mast cells are more commonly seen in indolent types of SM, whereas atypical type II mast cells and metachromatic blasts are more common in patients with mast cell leukemia and myelomastocytic leukemia; these latter disorders are associated with a poor prognosis and short survival.[6,7]

Histology

In most cases, histologic evaluation of a bone marrow biopsy, coupled with immunohistochemistry and/or special stains to identify mast cells, provides the best material to diagnose SM. The diagnostic criteria for SM include examination of tissue sections for multifocal aggregates of mast cells (see **Table 1**). Five patterns of bone marrow infiltration by mast cells are described.[8]

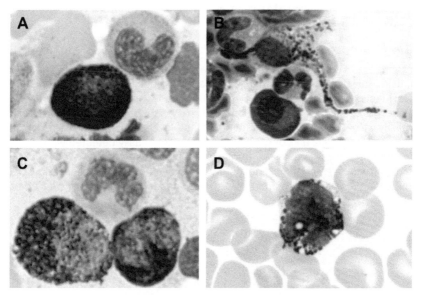

Fig. 1. Cytology of mast cells. (*A*) Typical mature tissue mast cell with well-granulated cytoplasm and a round to oval-shaped central nucleus adjacent to a band neutrophil. Basophils (not shown), in contrast, contain multilobated nuclei similar to a neutrophil. (*B*) Atypical mast cell type 1 with elongated cytoplasmic projections giving the cell a characteristic spindle shape containing reduced numbers of metachromatic granules. The nucleus is oval and eccentrically placed. (*C*) Two atypical mast cells type II with bilobed nuclei. Note the size of these atypical mast cells is larger than the adjacent neutrophil. (*D*) Metachromatic blast with high nuclear-to-cytoplasmic ratio, smooth chromatin, and scattered metachromatic granules from a patient with myelomastocytic leukemia. Bone marrow aspirate smears, Wright Giemsa stain, ×1000.

Pattern 1 is an *interstitial* pattern typically seen in mast cell hyperplasia (**Fig. 2**).

Patterns 2 through 4 involve *focal, dense infiltrates* of mast cells either alone (pattern 2) or coupled with additional interstitial mast cell components, located either preferentially around the focal infiltrates (pattern 3) or evenly distributed throughout the biopsy (pattern 4). Patterns 2, 3, and 4 characterize most SM cases (**Figs. 3** and **4**).

Pattern 5 represents *diffuse, dense* mast cell infiltrates that obliterate the marrow architecture, and is found in mast cell leukemia and smoldering SM (**Fig. 5**).

One type of focal, dense infiltrate is the *tryptase-positive compact round cell infiltrate of the bone marrow* (TROCI-BM) (**Fig. 6**). This particular pattern, while rare, brings the differential diagnosis of a specific set of myeloid neoplasms, including SM, mast cell leukemia, myelomastocytic leukemia, tryptase-positive acute myeloid leukemia, acute basophilic leukemia, and SM-AHNMD (**Table 4**).[9]

The dense infiltrates of mast cells in SM are typically perivascular and paratrabecular, formed by round or spindle-shaped mast cells and often accompanied by reticulin and collagen fibrosis (**Figs. 7** and **8**). Associated reactive lymphoid aggregates are quite common, as are accompanying eosinophils and plasma cells (**Figs. 9** and **10**). Immunophenotyping (flow cytometry, immunohistochemistry, and/or in situ hybridization) can separate reactive lymphocytes and polytypic plasma cells from their neoplastic counterparts. Osteosclerosis and an increase in small capillaries (neoangiogenesis) also can accompany mastocytosis (**Fig. 11**). Finally, in cases of SM-AHNMD, recognizing the mast cell infiltrate can be of particular challenge when the infiltrate is quite focal or masked by the non-mast neoplasm (**Fig. 12**). Approximately 20% to 30% of patients with SM will develop a second hematologic disease, which is usually a clonal myeloid disorder (**Fig. 13**).[9,10]

Ancillary Studies

Normal mast cells stain with chloracetate esterase, Giemsa, and toluidine blue, but the latter stain is pH dependent and these stains are less specific than immunophenotypic studies. Mast cells express CD33, CD43, CD68, CD117, and tryptase.[5] Tryptase is the most lineage specific of these markers, but may show high background staining, particularly in patients with high serum tryptase levels. Neoplastic mast cells also aberrantly express CD2 and/or CD25, with CD25 more easily detected with immunohistochemistry[11]; these markers are not present in normal or reactive mast cells. For practical purposes, an immunohistochemistry panel of CD117, tryptase, and CD25 is recommended to aid in confirming mast cell lineage and to identify an aberrant

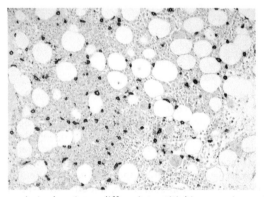

Fig. 2. Mast cell hyperplasia showing a diffuse interstitial increase in mast cells without any compact infiltrates (bone marrow biopsy, tryptase, ×200).

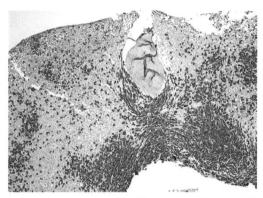

Fig. 3. Focal dense infiltrates of tryptase-positive mast cells around bone and vessels in a patient with SM and chronic myelomonocytic leukemia (bone marrow biopsy, tryptase, ×100).

immunophenotype. For flow cytometry, a panel containing CD117, CD45, CD2, and CD25 is helpful, although mast cells may be underrepresented in flow cytometry samples and difficult to identify.[12]

Point mutations of the tyrosine kinase receptor gene *KIT* are the most common genetic abnormality in mastocytosis and the most common mutation results in a substitution of valine for aspartate at codon 816 of exon 17, termed Asp816Val or D816 V. More than 95% of patients with SM have this mutation.[13] Other mutations have been described in exons 11 and 17.[14] *KIT* mutations are less common in pediatric and cutaneous mast cell tumors, and more than one-half of these mutations occur outside of exon 17.[15] *KIT* mutations are not specific for mastocytosis and do occur in other diseases.[16,17] Even the D816 V mutation is not disease specific, and for this reason, detection of the mutation represents only a minor diagnostic criterion (see **Table 1**). Molecular detection of *KIT* mutations can be performed on fresh bone marrow aspirate, clot sections or bone marrow biopsy sections; the latter should be fixed in formalin and decalcified in EDTA. Clot sections should be fixed in formalin. *KIT* mutation testing can be performed on peripheral blood if there are circulating mast cells or if the blood is involved by an AHNMD with the *KIT* mutation.

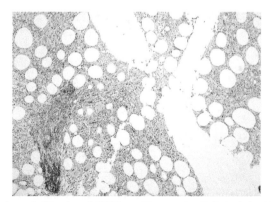

Fig. 4. Rare focal dense infiltrates of CD25-positive mast cells in indolent SM occupying less than 10% of marrow cellularity (bone marrow biopsy, CD25, ×100).

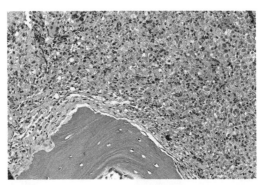

Fig. 5. Diffuse dense infiltrates of immature mast cells efface normal marrow architecture in mast cell leukemia (bone marrow biopsy, H&E, ×400).

Given the overlap in morphology between SM and myeloid and lymphoid neoplasms with eosinophilia and *PDGFRA* and *PDGFRB* abnormalities (**Fig. 14**), it may be necessary to perform additional analysis to exclude neoplasms with these molecular abnormalities, especially in cases of SM with a marked eosinophilia and loose networks of CD25+ mast cells. The *FIP1L1-PDGFRA* fusion is cryptic and thus conventional cytogenetic analysis is usually normal; fluorescence in situ hybridization (FISH) analysis or reverse transcriptase–polymerase chain reaction (RT-PCR) can be performed to detect this fusion gene.[18] In myeloid neoplasms with *PDGFRB* rearrangements, typically a t(5;12)(q31-q33;p12) is present on cytogenetic testing; nevertheless, molecular confirmation of the *ETV6-PDGFRB* fusion gene is helpful.[19] This distinction between SM and neoplasms with *PDGFRA* and *PDGFRB* abnormalities is vitally important, given the latter neoplasms' excellent response to imatinib,[18] in contrast to SM.

Differential Diagnosis

When increased mast cells are noted on smears or histologic sections, recognizing the cytology of the mast cells (normal, atypical type I, atypical type II, metachromatic blast) and the pattern of mast cell infiltration (interstitial, diffuse dense, focal dense, TROCI-BM) can direct the pathologist to a differential diagnosis (see **Figs. 1–6**).

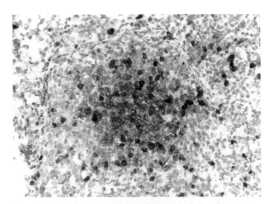

Fig. 6. Tryptase-positive compact round cell infiltrate of the bone marrow (TROCI-BM) in accelerated phase of chronic myeloid leukemia. These cells did not express CD117 (not shown) (bone marrow biopsy, tryptase, ×200).

Table 4
Differential diagnosis of systemic mastocytosis

Disease	Cell Pattern	Phenotype	KIT D816 V
Systemic mastocytosis	Compact, dense infiltrates meeting criteria for SM	Tryptase+, CD117+, CD25/CD2+[a]	+[b]
Acute basophilic leukemia	Interstitial	Tryptase weak+, CD117–/+, CD13/CD33+, 2D7+, BB1+, CD123+	–
Mast cell hyperplasia	Interstitial	Tryptase+, CD117+, CD25/CD2–	–
Myeloid neoplasms with eosinophilia and PDGFRA/PDGRFB abnormalities	Interstitial or clustered[c]	Tryptase+, CD117+, CD25+	–[d]
Myelomastocytic leukemia	Interstitial mast cells and blasts	Mast cells: tryptase+, CD117+, CD25/CD2– Blasts: CD34+, CD25–, CD117+	–
Tryptase-positive AML	Insterstitial	Tryptase+, CD117+, CD25–, CD34+, CD13/33+	–

Abbreviation: MC, mast cell.
 [a] Some cases of systemic mastocytosis may lack CD25/CD2 expression.
 [b] A small minority of cases lack the D816 V KIT mutation.
 [c] Mast cells may be scattered, in loose clusters, or cohesive clusters.
 [d] *FIP1L1-PDGFRA+* or *PDGFRB*-fusion variants.

Interstitial pattern (mast cell hyperplasia, mast cell leukemia, acute basophilic leukemia, tryptase-positive acute myeloid leukemia, myelomastocytic leukemia, myeloproliferative neoplasms with eosinophilia): Mast cell hyperplasia differs from the other neoplastic disorders by its normal mast cell cytology with small cell size, low nuclear-to-cytoplasm ratio, and round to oval nuclei. Histologically, reactive mast cells are increased in a loose scattered fashion without clusters or compact infiltrates (see **Fig. 2**). In contrast, mast cell leukemia will show sheets of mast cells,

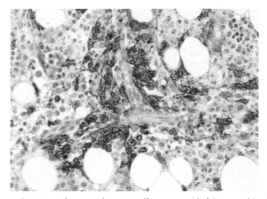

Fig. 7. Clusters of predominantly round mast cells surround this vessel in indolent SM (bone marrow biopsy, CD117, ×600).

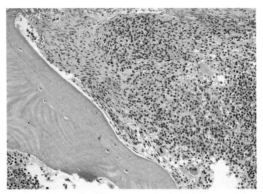

Fig. 8. Spindled mast cells comprise this paratrabecular aggregate in SM with adjacent clusters of reactive plasma cells (bone marrow biopsy, H&E, ×400).

typically with diffuse and focal dense areas, in addition to heavy interstitial infiltrates (see **Fig. 5**). On marrow smears, more than 20% of mast cells are detected and these are atypical, showing immature features including metachromatic blasts and/or atypical type II mast cells and criteria for SM are met. In the rare basophilic leukemia, the neoplastic cells are morphologically indistinguishable from the metachromatic blasts of mast cell leukemia, but these cells do not mark as true mast cells (low tryptase expression, CD117 negative) and express myeloid markers (CD13 and CD33) and CD123; thus, immunophenotyping "saves the day" in distinguishing acute basophilic leukemia from SM.[1] Tryptase-positive acute myeloid leukemia, another rare disorder, can also show a diffuse interstitial pattern in areas and shows strong tryptase expression, but lacks other features of mastocytosis; moreover, the cells cytologically resemble myeloblasts, usually of the M0 or M1 FAB subtype.[20] Myelomastocytic leukemia is a rare disease described in patients with advanced myeloid neoplasms (most commonly refractory anemia with excess blasts or acute myeloid leukemia [AML]) with elevated numbers of atypical mast cells who do not meet full criteria for SM. Typically there are greater than 5% myeloblasts and greater than 10% metachromatic blasts in the blood and/or marrow without focal dense mast cell infiltrates, without mast cell coexpression of CD2 or CD25, and without evidence of the D816 V KIT mutation (**Fig. 15**).[21] Myelomastocytic leukemia is a controversial entity

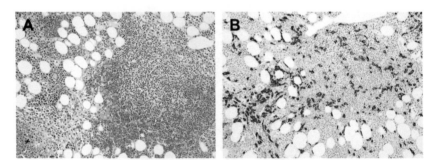

Fig. 9. A reactive lymphoid aggregate at right is adjacent to a loose collection of mast cells admixed with eosinophils in a case of indolent SM. Immunohistochemical staining for tryptase highlights a surprising number of clustered and single mast cells with cytoplasmic staining, including spindle forms. (A) H&E. (B) Tryptase. Bone marrow biopsy, ×500.

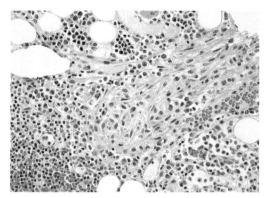

Fig. 10. The spindle-shaped mast cells in this aggregate are admixed with numerous eosinophils. On H&E sections, mast cell granules are not visible and the cytoplasm typically has a light eosinophilic color (bone marrow biopsy, ×600).

not widely recognized by pathologists and is not included in the 2008 WHO classification. In the myeloproliferative neoplasms associated with eosinophilia and *PDGFRA* abnormalities, loose aggregates of CD25+ spindled mast cells may be present in more than one-half of cases; CD25+ spindled mast cell infiltrates have also been described in myeloid neoplasms with *PDGFRB* abnormalities. However, criteria for SM are not fulfilled because the KIT D816 V mutation is absent and compact, dense mast cell infiltrates are lacking.[22]

Diffuse dense pattern (mast cell leukemia, smoldering SM): Although both mast cell leukemia and smoldering SM can show diffuse dense mast cell infiltrates in tissue sections with alteration of bone marrow architecture, as well as markedly elevated serum tryptase levels, mast cell leukemia exhibits "C findings," whereas smoldering SM does not.[1] Furthermore, mast cell leukemia shows marked atypia on cytologic smears, a feature that is lacking in smoldering SM.

Focal dense pattern (indolent SM, smoldering SM, well-differentiated SM, isolated bone marrow mastocytosis, mast cell hyperplasia, SM-AHNMD, aggressive SM): Although many types of SM can show focal dense mast cell infiltrates, one can

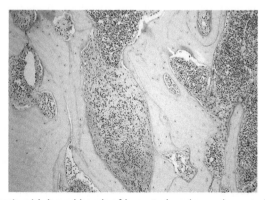

Fig. 11. Osteosclerosis with broad bands of bony trabeculae and paratrabecular collections of mast cells are present in this case of SM with associated chronic myelomonocytic leukemia (H&E, ×100).

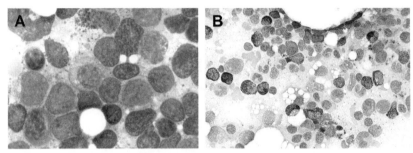

Fig. 12. (A) Acute myeloid leukemia with t(8;21)(q22;q22) was diagnosed in this bone marrow aspirate with sheets of blasts (Wright Giemsa, ×1000). (B) After induction chemotherapy, numerous atypical type II mast cells were unmasked (Wright Giemsa, ×600).

separate them into the more indolent disorders, aggressive SM, and SM-AHNMD. Rarely, mast cell hyperplasia may show focal dense mast cell infiltrates, but the mast cells lack atypia on smears and the cases do not fulfill criteria for SM. Indolent SM, the most common subtype of SM, shows focal dense mast cell infiltrates that minimally involve the bone marrow (<10% of marrow cellularity) with little effect on surrounding hematopoiesis; reactive lymphoid aggregates, plasmacytosis, and eosinophilia may be seen (see **Figs. 9** and **10**). The mast cells may be round or spindle shaped and skin lesions of urticaria pigmentosa are usually present (**Fig. 16**). Isolated bone marrow mastocytosis, smoldering SM, and well-differentiated mastocytosis all represent variants of indolent SM. In isolated bone marrow mastocytosis, there is no skin involvement and serum tryptase level is normal. Most of these cases were previously called *eosinophilic fibrohistiocytic bone marrow lesion.*[23] Smoldering SM has "B findings" and a greater degree of marrow infiltration than that seen in indolent SM (>30% of marrow cellularity) with a markedly elevated serum tryptase level. Well-differentiated SM is characterized by round mast cells with multifocal dense marrow infiltrates lacking CD25 and *KIT* D816 V mutation. A different, imatinib-sensitive *KIT* mutation has been described with this variant.[24] Aggressive SM has "C findings," atypical mast cells on smears and usually a markedly hypercellular marrow with focal dense and diffuse infiltration by atypical mast cells. Aggressive SM should be regarded as a diagnosis of exclusion because most cases are in fact SM-AHNMD when bone marrow and blood smears are carefully investigated. A variant of

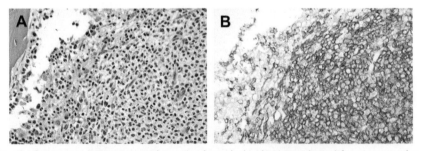

Fig. 13. Systemic mastocytosis with a mixed myelodysplastic/myeloproliferative neoplasm, unclassifiable. (A) Large aggregate of mast cells with clear cytoplasm and irregular nuclei admixed with eosinophils (H&E, ×400). (B) Crisp strong membrane staining with CD117 rings the mast cells (bone marrow biopsy, CD117, ×400).

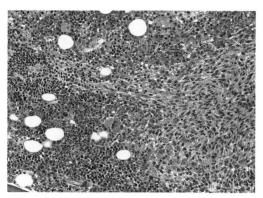

Fig. 14. Myeloid neoplasm with *PDGFRB* rearrangement and t(5;12). A compact clustered of spindled mast cells is present at right admixed with numerous eosinophils and fewer numbers of pigment-laden macrophages. At left an aggregate of lymphocytes is seen (H&E, ×200).

aggressive SM, lymphadenopathic mastocytosis with eosinophilia, has generalized lymphadenopathy and marked eosinophilia.[25]

TROCI-BM pattern (SM, mast cell leukemia, myelomastocytic leukemia, tryptase-positive AML, basophilic leukemia, SM-AHNMD): Tryptase-positive compact round cell infiltrates of the bone marrow raise a specific differential diagnosis requiring the

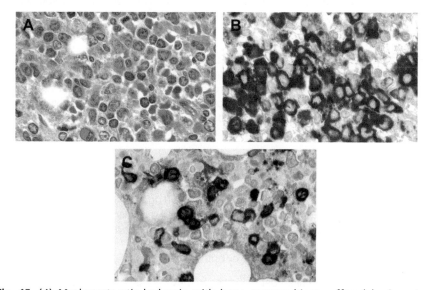

Fig. 15. (*A*) Myelomastocytic leukemia with bone marrow biopsy effaced by immature mononuclear cells (H&E, ×500). Discrete subsets of the immature cells stain strongly with myeloperoxidase (*B*) and tryptase (*C*), the latter in an interstitial pattern. Flow cytometry confirmed 2 populations of cells: myeloblasts and mast cells. The D816 V KIT mutation was absent and criteria for SM were not met. Circulating blasts and metachromatic blasts were also seen (not shown). (Images *courtesy of* Luke Shier, MD, University of Alberta Hospital, Edmonton, Canada. Case originally published in Arredondo A, Gotlib J, Shier L, et al. Myelomastocytic leukemia versus mast cell leukemia versus systemic mastocytosis associated with acute myeloid leukemia: a diagnostic challenge. Am J Hematol 2010;85:600–6.)

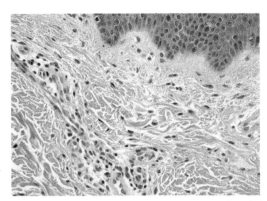

Fig. 16. A 27-year-old woman with urticaria pigmentosa and indolent SM. Histologic sections show a subtle superficial perivascular and interstitial infiltrate composed of mono-nuclear cells with pale eosinophilic cytoplasm (mast cells) and scattered eosinophils (skin, H&E, ×200).

application of lineage-specific markers to determine whether the neoplastic cells are mast cells or basophilic granulocytes (see **Fig. 6**).[9] In cases of SM and mast cell leukemia, expression of CD117 is found. In myelomastocytic leukemia and tryptase-positive AML, expression of CD34 and CD117 is found, whereas neither CD34 nor CD117 is detected in accelerated phases of chronic myeloid leukemia with numerous basophils ("basophilic leukemia"); basophil-related antigens such as 2D7 and CD123 are positive in the latter.

Diagnosis and Classification

In the 2008 WHO classification, SM is diagnosed when 1 major criterion and 1 minor criterion, or at least 3 minor criteria are present (see **Table 1**). The major diagnostic criterion for SM is fulfilled by the presence of multifocal dense mast cell infiltrates (≥15 mast cells per aggregate) detected histologically in the bone marrow or in another extracutaneous organ(s). Minor criteria include the following[2,3]:

1. Twenty-five percent or more of the mast cells in the infiltrate are spindle shaped or show atypical morphology, or 25% or more are immature or atypical on bone marrow aspirate smears.
2. Serum tryptase level is persistently greater than 20 ng/mL (note that this parameter is not valid if there is an associated clonal myeloid disorder).
3. The D816 V *KIT* mutation is detected in bone marrow, blood, or another extracuta-neous organ.
4. There is expression of CD2, CD25, or both in the neoplastic mast cells.

Indolent forms of systemic mast cell disease may be characterized by one or more "B findings" (see **Table 2**). If 2 or more "B findings" are present, the disease is classi-fied as smoldering SM. Treatment of mediator-related symptoms, when present, is commonly used in all SM variants, whereas cytoreductive agents are not prescribed. In contrast, aggressive SM and mast cell leukemia are characterized by 1 or more "C findings" (see **Table 2**); aggressive SM often requires cytoreductive therapy. In SM-AHNMD, WHO diagnostic criteria for both SM and a distinct non–mast cell hemato-logic neoplasm (such as a myelodysplastic syndrome, myeloproliferative neoplasm, acute leukemia, lymphoma, or plasma cell myeloma) are met.[7]

Mast cell leukemia is a rare subtype of SM characterized by leukemic spread of mast cells and an aggressive, rapidly progressing clinical course. By definition, mast cell leukemia meets criteria for SM with additional features, including (1) leukemic infiltration of the bone marrow and/or other extracutaneous organs by neoplastic mast cells, (2) at least 20% neoplastic mast cells in bone marrow and/or blood smears, and (3) high-grade cytologic findings.[2] "C findings" are commonly associated with mast cell leukemia.[26] Mast cell leukemia is the only advanced mastocytic disorder for which a cytologic diagnosis on an aspirate smear preparation is required to make the diagnosis.[27] To satisfy the major WHO criterion for SM, multifocal dense infiltrates in the bone marrow biopsy must be present, whereas mast cell leukemia is defined by diffuse and interstitial mast cell infiltrates.[2] Thus, the mast cell infiltrate in mast cell leukemia is dense and multifocal, but also has an additional diffuse component, representing a mixed pattern. Mast cells typically show marked atypia and often express CD25 and there are persistently elevated serum tryptase levels. In more than 50% of mast cell leukemia cases, the *KIT* mutation D816 V is detectable.

Prognosis

Prognosis in indolent SM is usually excellent and the course of the disease is typically benign. Advanced mast cell neoplasms such as aggressive SM and mast cell leukemia are notoriously difficult to manage and no curative treatments are currently available; the median survival time in mast cell leukemia is typically only 6 months. Patients should avoid triggers of mast cell activation, including exposure to extreme variations in temperature, excess exercise, and, in some patients, exposure to certain inciting drugs or alcohol. Treatment for advanced SM may include standard therapy to treat mediator symptoms,[7] along with cytoreductive therapy, such as interferon-α with or without corticosteroids, or cladribine in those who have slowly progressing aggressive SM.[5] However, major or partial responses are observed in only a subset of patients.[5,7] Rare patients have long-term survival after chemotherapy and bone marrow transplantation.[27,28] Importantly, the D816 V *KIT* mutation results in resistance to imatinib, thus this tyrosine kinase inhibitor is ineffective at treating SM.[29] Alternative tyrosine kinase inhibitors have shown some promise and clinical trials are ongoing.[30–32] SM-AHNMD is treated in a dichotomous fashion, with the AHNMD being treated independently of the SM, and vice versa[7] The prognosis of SM-AHNMD is typically driven by the AHNMD rather than the SM.

Pitfalls
Systemic Mastocytosis

! Mast cell nuclei are typically round to oval, whereas basophils have lobulated nuclei similar to neutrophils

! Paratrabecular and perivascular spindle-shaped cells may mimic fibrosis: check for mastocytosis using immunostains for CD117 and tryptase

! CD117 is not specific for mast cells, and may be seen in myeloblasts and proerythroblasts in the bone marrow

! Marrows with marked eosinophilia and loose collections of CD25+ mast cells could represent *PDGFRA/PDGFRB*-associated myeloid neoplasms; these patients will respond to imatinib, but patients with SM will not

ACKNOWLEDGMENTS

The authors would like to thank Daniel A. Arber, MD, for his help and advice.

REFERENCES

1. Horny HP. Mastocytosis: an unusual clonal disorder of bone marrow-derived hematopoietic progenitor cells. Am J Clin Pathol 2009;132(3):438–47.
2. Horny HP, Akin C, Metcalfe DD, et al. Mastocytosis. In: Swerdlow S, Campo E, Harris NL, et al, editors. WHO classification of tumours of haematopoietic and lymphoid tissues. Lyon (France). IARC Press; 2008. p. 53–63.
3. Valent P, Sperr WR, Schwartz LB, et al. Diagnosis and classification of mast cell proliferative disorders: delineation from immunologic diseases and non-mast cell hematopoietic neoplasms. J Allergy Clin Immunol 2004;114(1):3–11.
4. Horny HP, Parwaresch MR, Lennert K. Bone marrow findings in systemic mastocytosis. Hum Pathol 1985;16(8):808–14.
5. Horny HP, Sotlar K, Valent P. Mastocytosis: state of the art. Pathobiology 2007; 74(2):121–32.
6. Valent P, Samorapoompichi P, Sperr WR, et al. Myelomastocytic leukemia: myeloid neoplasm characterized by partial differentiation of mast cell-lineage cells. Hematol J 2002;3(2):90–4.
7. Valent P, Horny HP, Escribano L, et al. Diagnostic criteria and classification of mastocytosis: a consensus proposal. Leuk Res 2001;25(7):603–25.
8. Krokowski M, Sotlar K, Krauth MT, et al. Delineation of patterns of bone marrow mast cell infiltration in systemic mastocytosis: value of CD25, correlation with sub-variations of the disease and separation from mast cell hyperplasia. Am J Clin Pathol 2005;124(4):560–8.
9. Horny HP, Sotlar K, Stellmacher F, et al. The tryptase positive compact round cell infiltrate of the bone marrow (TROCI-BM): a novel histopathological finding requiring the application of lineage specific markers. J Clin Pathol 2006;59(3): 298–302.
10. Sperr WR, Horny HP, Lechner K, et al. Clinical and biological diversity of leukemias occurring in patients with mastocytosis. Leuk Lymphoma 2000;37(5–6): 473–86.
11. Sotlar K, Horny HP, Simonitsch I, et al. CD25 indicates the neoplastic phenotype of mast cells: a novel immunohistochemical marker for the diagnosis of systemic mastocytosis in routinely processed bone marrow biopsy specimens. Am J Surg Pathol 2004;28(10):1319–25.
12. Escribano L, Diaz-Agustin B, López A, et al. Immunophenotypic analysis of mast cells in mastocytosis: when and how to do it. Proposals of the Spanish network on mastocytosis (REMA). Cytometry B Clin Cytom 2004;58(1):1–8.
13. Garcia-Montero AC, Jara-Acevedo M, Teodosio C, et al. KIT mutation in mast cells and other bone marrow hematopoietic cell lineages in systemic mast cell disorders: a prospective study of the Spanish network on mastocytosis (REMA) in a series of 113 patients. Blood 2006;108(7):2366–72.
14. Feger F, Ribadeau DA, Lerich L, et al. Kit and c-kit mutations in mastocytosis: a short overview with special reference to novel molecular and diagnostic concepts. Int Arch Allergy Immunol 2002;127(2):110–4.
15. Bodemer C, Hermine O, Palmerini F, et al. Pediatric mastocytosis is a clonal disease associated with D816V and other activating c-KIT mutations. J Invest Dermatol 2010;130(3):804–15.

16. Lasota J, Miettinen M. Clinical significance of oncogenic KIT and PDGFRA mutations in gastrointestinal stromal tumours. Histopathology 2008;53(3):245–66.
17. Beghini A, Ripamonti CB, Cairoli R, et al. KIT activating mutations: incidence in adult and pediatric acute myeloid leukemia, and identification of an internal tandem duplication. Haematologica 2004;89(8):920–5.
18. Cools J, DeAngelo DJ, Gotlib J, et al. A tyrosine kinase created by fusion of the PDGFRA and FIP1L1 genes as a therapeutic target of imatinib in idiopathic hypereosinophilic syndrome. N Engl J Med 2003;348(13):1201–14.
19. Bain BJ, Fletcher SH. Chronic eosinophilic leukemias and the myeloproliferative variant of the hypereosinophilic syndrome. Immunol Allergy Clin North Am 2007;27(3):377–88.
20. Sperr WR, Jordan JH, Baghestanian M, et al. Expression of mast cell tryptase by myeloblasts in a group of patients with acute myeloid leukemia. Blood 2001; 98(7):2200–9.
21. Arredondo A, Gotlib J, Shier L, et al. Myelomastocytic leukemia versus mast cell leukemia versus systemic mastocytosis associated with acute myeloid leukemia: a diagnostic challenge. Am J Hematol 2010;85(8):600–6.
22. Pardanani A, Ketterling RP, Brockman SR, et al. CHIC2 deletion, a surrogate for FIP1L1-PDGFRA fusion, occurs in systemic mastocytosis associated with eosinophilia and predicts response to imatinib mesylate therapy. Blood 2003;102(9): 3093–6.
23. Rywlin AM, Hoffman EP, Ortega RS. Eosinophilic fibrohistiocytic lesion of bone marrow: a distinctive new morphologic finding, probably related to drug hypersensitivity. Blood 1972;40(4):464–72.
24. Akin C, Fumo G, Akif S, et al. A novel form of mastocytosis associated with a transmembrane c-kit mutation and response to imatinib. Blood 2004;103(8):3222–5.
25. Frieri M, Linn N, Schweitzer M, et al. Lymphadenopathic mastocytosis with eosinophilia and biclonal gammopathy. J Allergy Clin Immunol 1990;86(1):126–32.
26. Noack F, Sotlar K, Notter M, et al. A leukemic mast cell leukemia with abnormal immunophenotype and c-kit mutation D816V. Leuk Lymphoma 2004;45(11): 2295–302.
27. Valentini CG, Rondoni M, Pogliani EM, et al. Mast cell leukemia: a report of ten cases. Ann Hematol 2008;87(16):505–8.
28. Sperr WR, Drach J, Hauswirth AW, et al. Myelomastocytic leukemia: evidence for the origin of mast cells from the leukemic clone and eradication by allogeneic stem cell transplantation. Clin Cancer Res 2005;11(19 Pt 1):6787–92.
29. Ma Y, Zeng S, Metcalfe DD, et al. The c-KIT mutation causing human mastocytosis is resistant to STI571 and other KIT kinase inhibitors; kinases with enzymatic site mutations show different inhibitor sensitivity profiles than wild-type kinases and those with regulatory-type mutations. Blood 2002;99(5):1741–4.
30. Gotlib J, Berube C, Growney JD, et al. Activity of tyrosine kinase inhibitor PKC412 in a patient with mast cell leukemia with the D816V KIT mutation. Blood 2005; 106(8):2865–70.
31. Verstovsek S, Tefferi A, Cortes J, et al. Phase II study of dasatinib in Philadelphia chromosome-negative acute and chronic myeloid diseases, including systemic mastocytosis. Clin Cancer Res 2008;14(12):3906–15.
32. Ustun C, Corless CL, Savage N, et al. Chemotherapy and dasatinib induce long-term hematologic and molecular remission in systemic mastocytosis with acute myeloid leukemia with KIT D816V. Leuk Res 2009;33(5):735–41.

Diagnosis of Myelodysplastic Syndromes in Cytopenic Patients

Sa A. Wang, MD

KEYWORDS

- Cytopenia • Myelodysplastic syndromes • Flow cytometry
- Aplastic anemia • Cytogenetics • Algorithm
- Diagnostic criteria

OVERVIEW

Sustained ($\geq$6 months) clinical cytopenia involving one or more hematopoietic lineages (erythrocytes, neutrophils, or platelets) is a frequent laboratory finding in patients treated at ambulatory clinics and in hospitalized patients.[1–4] The first question to be addressed (usually by a clinician, before considering sampling the BM) is whether or not the cytopenia is due to decreased production of hematopoietic cells or increased destruction, consumption, or loss of blood cells. For cytopenia attributed to decreased production of hematopoietic cells, the underlying causes can be attributed to either an intrinsic hematopoietic stem cell disorder or secondary etiology. Increased destruction or consumption can be due to blood loss, hemolysis, hypersplenism, mechanical cardiac valve placement, and other factors. The current recommended guidelines for the initial clinical evaluation of patients with cytopenia generally include a review of the patient's medical history and a thorough laboratory work-up (complete blood count and assessment of iron, folate, and vitamin B_{12} levels). BM biopsies and aspirates are subsequently performed in some cases because of an unrevealing laboratory work-up or to rule out an infiltrative BM process.[3,4]

For pathologists who examine the BM, a diagnosis of cytopenia secondary to an infiltrative process (such as lymphoma, myeloma, or metastatic carcinoma) or an acute leukemia can usually be easily established based on morphologic evaluation and flow cytometry immunophenotyping (FCI). It can be more challenging, however, to establish a diagnosis of MDS, a clonal BM disorder characterized by peripheral

A version of this article originally appeared in *Surgical Pathology Clinics*, 3:4.
Department of Hematopathology, University of Texas, MD Anderson Cancer Center, Unit 72, 1515 Holcombe Boulevard, Houston, TX 77030-4009, USA
E-mail address: swang5@mdanderson.org

Hematol Oncol Clin N Am 25 (2011) 1085–1110
doi:10.1016/j.hoc.2011.09.009   hemonc.theclinics.com
0889-8588/11/$ – see front matter © 2011 Elsevier Inc. All rights reserved.

Pathologic Key Features of Myelodysplastic Syndromes

1. Myelodysplastic syndromes (MDS) are hematopoietic stem cell neoplasms that involve the blood and bone marrow (BM) and manifest with varying degrees of peripheral cytopenias and morphologic dysplasia.

2. The BM in MDS is often hypercellular with disturbed topography, but 15% of cases are hypocellular.

3. Morphologic dysplasia must be present in more than 10% of cells in at least one hematopoietic lineage; in the absence of significant dysplasia, MDS can only be diagnosed if characteristic cytogenetic abnormalities are present in the clinical setting of unremitting cytopenia.

4. Accurate enumeration of myeloblasts in MDS is critical for classification and risk stratification.

5. Flow cytometry immunophenotyping can be useful in differentiating a reactive process versus a neoplastic stem cell process, such as MDS.

---

cytopenia, ineffective hematopoiesis, morphologic dysplasia, and recurrent cytogenetic abnormalities. Traditionally, the gold standard for diagnosing MDS has been BM morphology and cytogenetic studies in conjunction with a clinical presentation of persistent and unexplained cytopenia.[5,6] Not all patients with clinically suspected MDS evince definitive morphologic dysplasia,[7–9] and some non-MDS-related cytopenias may mimic MDS on morphologic evaluation.[10] Moreover, cytogenetic abnormalities are infrequent in patients with MDS cases lacking excess blasts.[11] The 2008 World Health Organization (WHO) classification subcategorizes MDS into several different diseases, based on the types of cytopenias, morphology, and specific cytogenetic abnormalities. These disease categories have different clinical behaviors and prognosis. The MDS entities defined in the 2008 WHO classification and their abbreviations are listed in **Box 1**. Although there is no recognized pathologic grading scheme for MDS, for the purposes of this topic, lower-grade MDS cases are defined as blasts greater than 5%, including refractory cytopenia with unilineage dysplasia (RCUD), refractory cytopenia with multilineage dysplasia (RCMD), and MDS with

---

Box 1
Myelodysplastic syndrome entities according to the WHO 2008 classification

Refractory cytopenia with unilineage dysplasia (RCUD)

    Refractory neutropenia

    Refractory anemia

    Refractory thrombocytopenia

Refractory anemia with ring sideroblasts (RARS)

Refractory cytopenia with multilineage dysplasia (RCMD)

Refractory anemia with excess blasts (RAEB)

    RAEB-1

    RAEB-2

MDS with isolated del(5q) abnormality

MDS, unclassified

Therapy-related MDS (t-MDS)

del(5q), whereas higher-grade MDS cases are defined as blast greater than or equal to 5%, including refractory anemia with excess blasts (RAEB).

Diagnosing MDS can be particularly challenging in patients who have received chemotherapy for primary malignancies and developed prolonged cytopenia. In such patients, a question to answer is whether the cytopenia is attributed to BM injury due to exogenous factors or if MDS has developed secondary to the chemotherapy. Morphologic dysplasia is a frequent finding in postchemotherapy BM samples and becomes less reliable in making the distinction between MDS and postchemotherapy BM injury. A similarly challenging situation exists in the differential diagnosis between aplastic anemia (AA) and hypoplastic MDS cases. Although the BM of patients with AA exhibits hypocellularity and usually lacks significant dysplasia,[12] in some cases the distinction between hypocellular MDS and AA may not be possible.[9,13] Morphologic evaluation can be further hampered by suboptimal BM material. For example, core biopsy samples may be of inadequate length, consist predominantly of cortical bone, or exhibit obscuring crush artifact. In addition, aspirate smears may be inadequate because of hemodilution, air drying, or poor staining.

This content addresses the diagnostic challenges faced by pathologists interpreting BM samples taken to evaluate cytopenic patients. The morphologic and clinical features that distinguish MDS from cytopenias secondary to non-MDS causes are described, in particular, the appropriate interpretation of cytogenetic findings and application of ancillary testing (mainly FCI). An algorithm based on the WHO and International Working Group (IWG) guidelines for diagnosis of MDS is also provided.

CLINICAL FEATURES

As defined by the International Prognostic Scoring System (IPSS) for MDS, cytopenia is characterized by a hemoglobin level less than 10 g/dL, absolute neutrophil count less than 1.8×10^9/L, and platelet count less than 100×10^9/L.[14] The IWG defines cytopenia as a hemoglobin level less than 11 g/dL, absolute neutrophil count less than 1.5×10^9/L, and platelet count less than 100×10^9/L.[15] Cytopenia in MDS is often unremitting or progressive. In some patients, however, cytopenia can be less severe at presentation or have less than a 6-month duration due to early detection. A diagnosis of MDS can still be rendered in such settings if definitive morphologic and/or cytogenetic findings are present (**Box 2**).[15,16]

Most patients with MDS present with cytopenia-related symptoms. Symptoms related to anemia, such as fatigue and malaise, with eventual transfusion dependence, are most common. Patients can also present with petechiae, ecchymoses, and nose and gum bleeding due to thrombocytopenia. Fever, cough, or septic shock may be manifestations of serious bacterial or fungal infections secondary to neutropenia. Hepatosplenomegaly or lymphadenopathy is uncommon in MDS patients. Therapy-related MDS (t-MDS) and other therapy-related myeloid neoplasms secondary to alkylating agents and/or ionizing radiation most commonly occur 5 to 10 years after exposure. Patients often present with t-MDS and evidence of BM failure, although a minority may present with t-MDS/myeloproliferative neoplasm (MPN) or with overt therapy-related acute myeloid leukemia (AML). Therapy-related myeloid neoplasms after treatment with topoisomerase II inhibitors have a latency period of approximately 1 to 5 years; most of these patients do not develop MDS but instead present with overt AML. In practice, many patients have received chemotherapeutic regimens that include both alkylating agents and topoisomerase II inhibitors and the clinicopathologic features may not be clear-cut. In addition, in elderly patients who receive cytotoxic therapy, cytopenias may be due to coincidental primary MDS or concurrent

---

Box 2
Minimal diagnostic criteria for patients with myelodysplastic syndromes, as recommended by the International Working Conference (2007)

A. Prerequisite criteria (both 1 and 2 required)

   1. Constant cytopenia in one or more of the following cell lineages:
      - Erythroid (hemoglobin <11 g/dL[a])
      - Neutrophilic (absolute neutrophil count <1.5 × 10^9/L[b]) or
      - Megakaryocytic (platelets <100 × 10^9/L)

   2. Exclusion of all other hematopoietic or nonhematopoietic disorders as the primary reason for cytopenia/dysplasia

B. MDS-related decisive criteria (at least one required)

   - Dysplasia in ≥10% of all cells in at least one of the following lineages in the BM smear: erythroid, neutrophilic, or megakaryocytic, or >15% ringed sideroblasts (iron stain)
   - 5%–19% Blast cells in the BM or PB
   - Typical chromosomal abnormality (by conventional karyotyping or fluorescence in situ hybridization [FISH])

C. Co-criteria (for patients fulfilling "A" but not any of the "B" criteria above and who otherwise show typical clinical features [eg, transfusion-dependent macrocytic anemia]) (at least one required)

   - Abnormal phenotype of BM cells clearly indicative of a monoclonal population of erythroid and/or myeloid cells, determined by flow cytometry,
   - Clear molecular signs of a monoclonal cell population on X-inactivation assay, gene chip profiling, or point mutation analysis (eg, *RAS* mutations),
   - Markedly and persistently reduced colony formation (±cluster formation) of BM and/or circulating progenitor cells by colony-forming unit assay.

[a] The WHO 2008 classification recommends using a hemoglobin level of <10 g/dL.
[b] The WHO 2008 classification recommends using an absolute neutrophil count level of <1.8 × 10^9/L.

MDS due to genetic predisposition to cancer. Nevertheless, because they are difficult or impossible to distinguish from t-MDS, according to the WHO classification such cases are considered by default to represent t-MDS.

DIAGNOSIS: MICROSCOPIC FEATURES
Peripheral Blood

The peripheral blood (PB) in patients with MDS nearly always shows some evidence of cytopenia. In addition, the anemia is often macrocytic and the red cell distribution width is often increased. Patients with significant ring sideroblasts (RS) in the marrow may show a dimorphic red cell appearance due to a combination of macrocytes and hypochromic microcytes. Granulocytic dysplasia may be more visible in the PB than in the BM. Recognizing and reporting circulating blasts are important, because the presence of these blasts can change the disease classification and predict patients' clinical outcomes. Circulating immature cells, including blasts, can also be seen in patients who have received growth factor treatment, in those with an actively regenerating BM, in those with an acute marrow stress such as sepsis, or in those who have undergone recent stem cell transplantation.

Bone Marrow Biopsy

Bone marrow biopsy is important for assessing cellularity, relative lineage proportions, fibrosis, stromal alterations, and megakaryocytic dysplasia. Normal BM usually shows a cellularity appropriate for a patient's age, with orderly maturation and a normal cellular distribution: the myeloid precursors are generally found along the bone trabeculae, whereas the erythroid and megakaryocytic precursors are located more centrally (**Fig. 1**A). In MDS, the BM is usually hypercellular, and the BM topography is disrupted (see **Fig. 1**B). Altered stroma is common, including markedly uneven distribution of fat cells with alteration of adipocyte size, increased histiocytes, increased small blood vessels, and increased reticulin fibrosis. Significant differences in the size of hemopoietic islands are often present and the erythroid islands may be disrupted or poorly delineated. Abnormal localization of immature precursors (ALIPs), defined as clusters or aggregates of myeloblasts and promyelocytes located away from bone trabeculae (see **Fig. 1**C), is an adverse prognostic feature in MDS and is an uncommon finding in lower-grade MDS cases.[17] However, ALIPs are not unique to MDS and can be seen in active BM regeneration or after growth factor treatment.[18,19]

Immunohistochemistry (IHC) can be useful in assessing for MDS, especially in a case of fibrotic or hypocellular BM. The expression of CD34, a marker of early progenitor cells, is positive in most MDS blasts, regardless of the MDS subtype.[20]

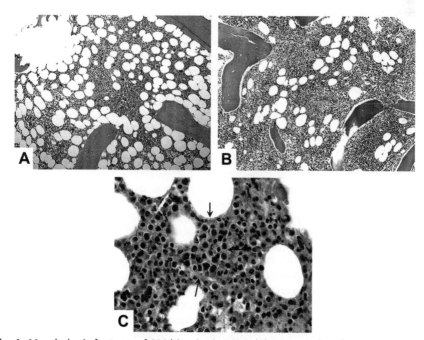

Fig. 1. Morphologic features of BM biopsies in MDS. (*A*) Topography of normal BM shows a normal cellular distribution, with preserved erythroid islands and normal appearing megakaryocytes. (*B*) Altered BM topography in a patient with MDS: the marrow is hypercellular, with altered cellular distribution, increased histiocytes, and increased vasculature. Dysplastic megakaryocytes are present, and appreciated at this power. (*C*) Abnormal localization of immature precursors (ALIPs), clusters of large immature cells (*arrows*) located away from the bone trabecula are present. The cellular components of ALIPs are mainly composed of myeloblasts and promyelocytes.

The presence of increased and/or clustered CD34+ blasts not only helps confirm a diagnosis of MDS but also assists in identifying ALIPs that are correlated with increased risk of transformation to AML.[21] CD34 is also present on endothelium and sinus lining cells, highlighting the increased angiogenesis characteristic of MDS. In rare cases, blasts in MDS are negative for CD34 and CD117 (c-KIT) may be used as an alternative blast marker; however, CD117 also stains some early erythroid precursors (pronormoblasts), some promyelocytes, and mast cells. Megakaryocytic markers, such as CD61, CD42b, and von Willebrand factor-associated protein, are useful for highlighting micromegakaryocytes and abnormal groupings or clusterings of megakaryocytes. These markers are also helpful in differentiating MDS from acute megakaryocytic leukemia (M7), where the megakaryoblasts have an immature phenotype, most commonly CD61+ but with partial or negative staining for CD42 and von Willebrand factor-associated protein.

Bone Marrow Aspirate

High-quality BM aspirate smears are critical for diagnosing and classifying MDS. BM aspirate evaluation includes recording the percentage of blasts and the degree of unilineage or multilineage dysplasia. Dysplasia must be present in at least 10% of the cells of any lineage, and the particular dysplastic changes seen may be relevant in predicting the biology and specific cytogenetic abnormalities of MDS.

Dysgranulopoiesis includes nuclear hypolobation, such as the pseudo-Pelger-Huët anomaly, hypersegmentation of the nuclei at an inappropriate stage, and abnormal cytoplasm ix granularity (agranularity, hypogranularity, hypergranularity or large, irregularly shaped eosinophilic pseudo-Chédiak-Higashi granules). Abnormally large or small granulocytes are also evidence of dysplasia, but giant neutrophils with nuclear hypersegmentation can also be seen in patients with vitamin B_{12} or folate deficiency. Dysplastic features present at earlier stages of myeloid lineage include hypogranulation, abnormally shaped (eg, elongated) granules, abnormal nuclear lobation, and nuclear/cytoplasmic dyssynchrony (**Fig. 2**A, B). Recognization of dysplastic features in early myeloid cells is important, especially in cases of MDS with left-shifted myeloid maturation.

Dyserythropoietic features include nuclear budding, internuclear bridging, karyorrhexis, multinuclearity, nuclear hyperlobation, cytoplasmic basophilic stippling, and vacuoles. Megaloblastoid change (nuclear-cytoplasmic dyssynchrony) is nonspecific and is common in non-MDS BM samples, thus should not be overinterpreted. RS, another manifestation of dyserythropoiesis, should have at least five siderotic granules present, covering at least one-third of the circumference of the nucleus.[5,22] Erythroblasts with less than five granules or with granules that are not in a perinuclear location should not be counted as RS. The presence of 15% RS or greater in a BM with less than 5% blasts classify patients as having refractory anemia with RS (RARS) if dysplasia is confined to the erythroid lineage. The presence of RS in MDS with multilineage dysplasia, cases with specific cytogenetic abnormalities, or those with increased blasts (5% or greater) do not change the MDS subcategorization. RS may occur in non-neoplastic conditions, such as alcoholism, hereditary sideroblastic anemia, and due to effects of certain drugs.

Marked erythroid hyperplasia (50% or greater) with or without left-shifted erythroid maturation (see **Fig. 2**C) can be seen in approximately 15% of patients with MDS. RS are frequently present (see **Fig. 2**D). In these patients, myeloblasts should be assessed as a proportion of nonerythroid cells: if myeloblasts are 20% or greater of nonerythroid cells, the case would meet criteria for acute erythroid leukemia, erythroid/myeloid subtype (FAB: AML-M6A); if myeloblasts are less than 20% of

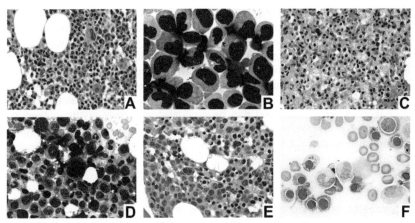

Fig. 2. Unusual features that can be seen in some cases of MDS. (*A*) MDS with myeloid hyperplasia and left-shifted myeloid maturation in the bone marrow biopsy; also present in the field are dysplastic megakaryocytes. (*B*) Myeloid lineage dysplasia can be observed in early and intermediate stage myeloid cells in the bone marrow aspirate. (*C*) MDS with pure red cell aplasia (BM biopsy). Unusual features that can be seen in some cases of MDS. (*D*) MDS with erythroid hypoplasia. The rare erythroid cells present are mainly immature forms (BM aspirate). (*E, F*) Erythroid-predominant MDS case with left-shifted erythroid maturation on the bone marrow biopsy (*E*) and numerous RS on iron stain (*F*); such cases should not be misdiagnosed as pure erythroidleukemia (AML M6B).

nonerythroid cells, the current recommendation is to enumerate the blasts as a proportion of total cells for subcategorization. Recent studies have shown that in erythroid-predominant MDS, however, blast calculation as a proportion of BM nonerythroid cells may be better than total nucleated cells for stratifying patients into prognostically relevant groups,[23,24] and MDS with erythroid predominance and M6A may be a biologic continuum that is arbitrarily divided by a blast cut-off.[23] Conversely, erythroid hypoplasia or aplasia is observed in approximately 5% of MDS cases (see **Fig. 2**E, F) and is often associated with an oligo- or monoclonal T-cell proliferation,[25] suggesting immune-mediated destruction of erythroid precursors. Some of these patients may respond to cyclosporine treatment.[26]

Dysmegakaryopoiesis in MDS is characterized by micromegakaryocytes with hypolobated nuclei; megakaryocytes of all sizes with monolobated nuclei; or megakaryocytes with multiple, widely separated nuclei (pawn-ball appearance). However, the latter forms can be seen in non-MDS conditions, such as paraneoplastic syndrome. Megakaryocytes can be increased, decreased, or normal in number. In evaluating megakaryocyte dysplasia, the best approach is to make the initial evaluation based on BM biopsy and then verify the findings on the BM aspirate smears. Commenting on dysmegakaryopoiesis should be based on an assessment of at least 20 to 30 megakaryocytes, ideally including evaluation of megakaryocytes in both the biopsy sections and aspirate smears.

Blast recognition and enumeration are critical in the diagnosis, risk stratification, and assessment of treatment response in MDS. A 500-cell differential count is required for accurate blast enumeration. The presence of Auer rods shifts the classification to RAEB-2, regardless of the blast percentage. Myeloblasts in MDS often show marked heterogeneity in size and can be classified into two morphologic types: agranular and granular. Promyelocytes in MDS can be misinterpreted as granular blasts due to dysplastic changes. Normal promyelocytes have a visible Golgi zone, uniformly dispersed azurophilic granules, and, in most instances, basophilic cytoplasm, whereas dysplastic promyelocytes may have reduced or irregular cytoplasmic basophilia, a poorly developed Golgi zone, hyper- or hypogranularity, or irregular distribution (clumps) of granules. Unlike most blasts in MDS, however, dysplastic promyelocytes should still contain an oval or indented nucleus that is often eccentric with somewhat coarse chromatin and at least a faintly visible Golgi zone. Dysplastic promyelocytes are also often larger than myeloblasts.[22] Some myeloblasts can have deeply basophilic cytoplasm and can be confused with early erythroid precursors (**Fig. 3**). Erythroid precursors have relatively mature clumped chromatin and often larger than myeloblasts at early stages.

DIAGNOSIS: ANCILLARY STUDIES
Flow Cytometric Immunophenotyping

Flow cytometric immunophenotyping (FCI) is a highly sensitive and reproducible method for quantitatively and qualitatively evaluating hematopoietic cell abnormalities. FCI abnormalities in MDS have been shown to be highly correlated with morphologic dysplasia and cytogenetic abnormalities.[27–29] In addition, FCI is less subjective and may be more sensitive and less affected by specimen quality than morphologic evaluation of dysplasia on smears. In particular, FCI demonstrates usefulness in supporting or ruling out MDS in the most diagnostically challenging BM samples obtained from patients with chronic, persistent cytopenia with no significant morphologic dysplasia or cytogenetic abnormalities.[30,31] A positive FCI result is more indicative of MDS or MDS/MPN whereas a negative FCI result is more frequently associated with non-MDS-related cytopenia. The use of FCI as an ancillary test in diagnosing MDS is gradually gaining acceptance by most pathologists. Given the wide range of findings observed in MDS thus far, however, FCI is only recommended for experienced laboratories, because some of the changes seen in FCI overlap with the changes seen in reactive and recovering BM samples.

Recently, the European LeukemiaNet has published standardization of FCI in diagnosis of MDS, providing guidelines on panel design and data interpretation.[32] Most published studies using FCI for diagnosing MDS are based on interpreting altered myelomonocytic differentiation or maturation patterns, using antigen combinations, such as CD13/CD16, CD11b/CD16, CD64/CD10, CD33/HLA-DR, CD65, and CD15.

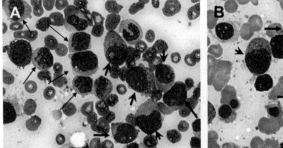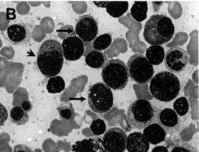

Fig. 3. Myeloblasts in MDS can be difficult to differentiate from dysplastic promyelocytes and dysplastic erythroid elements (*A, B*). Long thick arrows point to blasts. Note that one blast panel shows basophilic cytoplasm reminiscent of a pronormoblast, but contains a single centrally located nucleolus and dispersed chromatin and is smaller than a pronormoblast. Short thick arrows point to dysplastic promyelocytes with ill-defined Golgi zones and round or indented nuclei. Thin arrows point to dysplastic monocytes.

These approaches are sensitive, and MDS cases have demonstrated multiple abnormalities on FCI. However, myelomonocytic maturation patterns on FCI can show alterations in patients with reactive conditions, such as in patients with regenerating BM, those who have received growth factor treatment, and those with acute BM injury, severe infection, HIV, or autoimmune conditions. In addition, specimen quality such as hemodilution, or aged samples as well as increased eosinophils, can alter some normal patterns and the expression levels of some markers (eg, CD16, CD11b, and CD10). Moreover, abnormalities of some markers, such as decreased CD33 expression, can be attributed to genetic polymorphism and are not necessarily indicative of dysplasia. Although these nonspecific changes can be recognized,[28] the pattern recognition methodology requires that pathologists have extensive knowledge and experience in normal myelomonocytic maturation patterns and understand the immunophenotypic mimics.

In contrast, a focus on myeloblast phenotype seems to be a better approach.[20,31,33] Changes in myeloblasts more reliably indicate a stem cell neoplasm and are uncommonly seen in reactive conditions. These findings are easier for pathologists to interpret and report. This type of FCI analytic approach is focused on CD34+ cells, which in a reactive BM should show diverse differentiation and maturation patterns (**Fig. 4**). On side scatter versus CD45, normal myeloid precursors are scattered, showing a normal level

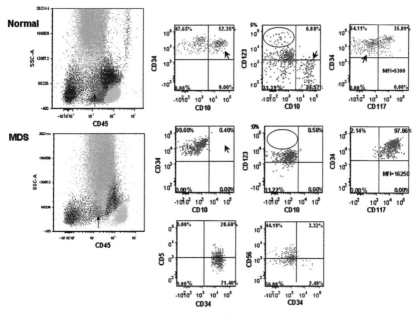

Fig. 4. FCI of MDS using an approach focusing on CD34+ cells. The upper row shows a normal marrow (lymphoma staging). Side scatter versus CD45 shows normal granularity of myeloid cells, well-separated myeloid (*light green*) and monocytic (*dark blue*) populations, with many hematogones and normal CD45 expression level of CD34+ myeloid precursors (red, *arrow*). The CD34+ cells contain many CD10+ hematogones (*short arrow*), CD123+ plasmacytoid dendritic precursors (*circled*), and myeloblasts with a normal CD117 expression level. The lower rows show BM from a patient with MDS. Side scatter versus CD45 shows hypogranulation of maturing myeloid cells (*light green*) and decreased CD45 expression on CD34+ blasts (*arrow*) and monocytes (*dark blue*). The CD34+ compartment is devoid of hematogones (*short arrow*) and plasmacytoid dendritic precursors (*circled*), and shows increased CD117 expression as well as aberrant expression of CD5 and CD56 (*bottom panels*).

of CD45 expression (often at the same level of granulocytes and side scatter). The normal CD34+ stem cells are able to produce hematogones (normal CD19+, CD10+ immature B-cell precursors), plasmacytoid dendritic precursors (CD123bright+, HLA-DR+), differentiating myeloid precursors (CD34+, CD15+, CD65+), and monocytic precursors (CD34+, CD64+, CD4+). In contrast, the CD34+ blasts in MDS appear to be clonal, forming a discrete population on side scatter versus CD45 and lacking evidence of differentiation toward hematogones, plasmacytoid dendritic cells, or monocytes. Alterations of antigenic expression levels, such as decreased or increased CD45 expression, increased CD34 or CD117 expression (see **Fig. 4**), increased CD33 or CD13 expression, or decreased CD38 expression, are often observed. Aberrant expression of lymphoid antigens (eg, CD2, CD5, CD7, and CD56) can also be observed.

The FCI analysis based on CD34+ blasts can be combined with significant changes in myelomonocytic cells to improve detection sensitivity and specificity. These changes include marked hypogranulation of granulocytes, significant alterations or asynchronous maturation of myelomonocytic cells, and substantial expression of CD56 on maturing granulocytes or monocytes. Examples of the markers and antibody combinations for MDS on FCI are shown in **Table 1**. Changes observed in CD34+ blasts and myelomonocytic cells from MDS cases are shown in **Box 3**. A positive FCI result does not distinguish MDS from MDS/MPN or some cases of MPN: some MPN, especially chronic idiopathic myelofibrosis, can exhibit similar changes as MDS. FCI abnormalities alone are not considered sufficient to diagnose MDS in the 2008 WHO Classification of Tumours of Haematopoietic and Lymphoid Tissue; however, it is recommended that cases with borderline dysplasia and no cytogenetic abnormalities but FCI results highly suggestive of MDS be re-evaluated over several months for definitive morphologic or cytogenetic evidence of MDS.

Although FCI is useful at demonstrating aberrant phenotypes of blasts and differentiating cells in MDS, it is not recommended as a method of enumerating blasts. Not all

Table 1
Examples of flow cytometric panels for myelodysplastic syndromes (focusing on the blast population)

4-Color Panel	5-Color Panel	6- and 7-Color Panel
Chromogens: FITC, PE, PerCPCy5.5, APC	Chromogens: FITC, PE, ECD, PEcy5.5, PEcy7	Chromogens: FITC, PE, PerCPCy5.5, PEcy7, APC, V500, V450
CD45, CD10, CD34, CD117	CD38, CD10, CD45, CD117, CD34	CD65, CD64, CD34, CD10, CD2, CD45, CD14
CD15, CD56, CD34, CD33	CD15, CD56, CD45, CD33, CD34	
CD7, CD2, CD34, CD5	CD7, CD2, CD45, CD5, CD34	CD7, CD5, CD34, CD38, CD45, CD19
HLA-DR, CD38, CD34, CD123	HLA-DR, CD38, CD45, CD123, CD34	HLA-DR, CD123, CD34, CD10, CD184, CD45, CD56
CD16, CD11b, CD45, CD13	CD16, CD11b, CD45, CD13, CD34	CD16, CD11b, CD34, CD33, CD13, CD45, CD15
CD14, CD64, CD45, HLA-DR	CD14, CD64, CD45, HLA-DR, CD34	
Kappa, Lambda, CD45, CD19	Kappa, Lambda, CD19, CD45, CD5	Kappa, Lambda, CD19, CD20, CD5, CD45
CD8, CD4, CD45, CD3	CD8, CD57, CD45, CD3, CD4	CD57, CD4, CD3, CD8, CD45, CD56

Box 3
Antigenic abnormalities detected on flow cytometry in patients with myelodysplastic syndromes

CD34+ blasts

- Decreased numbers or absence of hematogones and plasmacytoid dendritic precursors
- Discrete population formed
- Increased CD117 and CD34 expression
- Decreased or increased CD45 expression
- Increased CD33 and CD13 expression
- Increased CD123 expression
- Aberrant expression of CD2, CD5, CD7, and CD56
- Decreased CD38 expression
- Absent or markedly increased CD15, CD64, and CD65 expression
- Aberrant CD10 and CD19 expression (make sure they are not hematogones)
- Increased in numbers ($\geq$3%)

Maturing myeloid cells[a]

- Hypogranulation
- CD11b/CD13/CD16 abnormalities
- Decreased CD33, CD15, and CD65 expression
- Decreased CD38 expression and increased HLA-DR expression
- Decreased CD64 expression on relative immature population (no granulocytes)
- Decreased or absence of CD10 expression on granulocytes
- CD56 expression (>15%)
- Aberrant expression of CD2, CD5, CD7, and CD56

Monocytes[a]

- Decreased CD45 expression
- Decreased or increased CD64 expression, decreased CD14 expression
- Decreased HLA-DR expression, increased CD184 expression
- Decreased CD13 expression
- Decreased CD11b expression
- Loss of CD16 expression
- Increased CD15 and CD65 expression
- CD56 expression (>25%)
- Aberrant CD2, CD5, and CD7 expression

[a] Abnormalities identified in CD34+ blasts are more specific for a stem cell neoplasm whereas changes on maturing myelomonocytic cells are relatively nonspecific, especially in patients who have received chemotherapy and growth factor treatment and who have acute illness.

myeloblasts express CD34, and not all CD34+ cells are myeloblasts (for example, early hematogones are CD34+). Furthermore, the number of blasts enumerated on FCI can be affected by hemodilution, incomplete red blood cell lysis, lysis of late-stage nucleated red blood cells, suboptimal cell viability due to sample aging, and cell loss due to sample processing. Often, FCI underestimates the blasts compared with morphologic counting or IHC performed on the BM biopsy. When a BM sample shows marked erythroid hyperplasia, the blasts detected on FCI may be overestimated because of erythroid lysis.

Cytogenetics

Conventional karyotyping remains an essential component of the diagnostic work-up of any patient with suspected MDS, but these results need to be interpreted with caution. Isolated (nonclonal) cytogenetic abnormalities are commonly observed in BM samples and may represent an artifact of short-term culture before harvesting. To avoid false-positive results, a standardized definition for clonality, such as finding the same chromosomal gain or structural aberration in at least two BM cells and the same chromosome loss in at least three BM cells, is essential. In borderline cases or in the post-treatment setting where low numbers of metaphases are obtained, confirmation of the suspected chromosome changes by FISH on interphase (noncultured) cells is recommended. Clonal cytogenetic abnormalities are observed in approximately 50% of MDS cases and include many different alterations: a recent multicenter study showed 684 different types of chromosome abnormalities among 1080 patients with MDS who had abnormal karyotypes.[34] The IPSS uses cytogenetic abnormalities to define three risk categories: (1) good, which includes a normal karyotype, isolated interstitial del(5q), isolated del(20q), and −Y; (2) poor, which includes a complex karyotype with more than three abnormalities, as well as del(7q) and −7, either alone or in combination with other anomalies; and (3) intermediate, which includes all other abnormalities.[14] Recent studies have shown that some of the less common cytogenetic abnormalities seen in MDS may have different roles in terms of clinical outcome from their IPSS assignment, suggesting that a more sophisticated classification scheme is needed.[34–36] In addition, as therapy shifts, additional evaluations of these cytogenetic risk associations will be required. One such attempt at improving the IPSS scoring identified additional favorable cytogenetic results as del(12 p), del(9 p), +21, −21, del(11 p), del(15 p), and del(11q); reclassified sole del(7q) as intermediate risk; and added i(17q) and other forms of 17p loss as poor-risk changes.[37]

Fluorescence in Situ Hybridization

FISH has also been used to evaluate MDS cases for recurring genetic abnormalities.[36–38] MDS FISH panels include probes for detection of −5/del(5q), −7/del(7q), del(20q), and trisomy 8. The major advantage of FISH is its relatively high sensitivity with regard to the number of scorable cells as compared with the routine analysis of only 20 cells by conventional cytogenetics. FISH can be informative in MDS cases with karyotype failure as well as in cases of RAEB and RCMD showing a normal G-band karyotype.[38] FISH has been shown to have only limited usefulness in cases of RCUD and in MDS cases that have abnormal karyotypes by conventional cytogenetics.[39] In addition, the clinical relevance of low percentages of abnormal cells which are near the cut-off value in FISH assays remains unclear, apart from residual disease detection in patients with a previously characterized abnormality. In particular, the precision for detecting deletions varies with the probe used, and small populations that represent less than 6% to 8% of the total number of cells may fall beneath the threshold of detection for the assay.[40]

Comparative Genomic Hybridization Arrays and Single-nucleotide Polymorphism Arrays

Comparative genomic hybridization arrays[41,42] and single-nucleotide polymorphism arrays[43,44] are potential complementary techniques that can be applied to detect unbalanced chromosomal rearrangements in MDS interphase cells. When applied and interpreted together with conventional karyotyping and FISH, these arrays can improve the diagnostic yield for identifying genetic abnormalities in MDS and can better describe abnormal karyotypes. The clinical impact of alterations found by single-nucleotide polymorphism array or comparative genomic hybridization array, however, is still a subject of intense research.

Molecular Testing

Molecular clonality assays (such as G6PD isoenzymes, restriction-linked polymorphisms, and X-linked DNA polymorphisms of the androgen receptor gene) have helped to define MDS as a clonal disorder but are rarely used in clinical practice. In contrast, molecular genetic analyses looking for mutations and copy number changes in oncogenes and tumor suppressor genes are more informative as to the pathogenesis of MDS. Following the model used for AML, such mutations have been grouped as class I, where they target genes involved in signal transduction (commonly *FLT3*, *RAS* genes, and *KIT*), or as class II, where they involve transcription factors affecting differentiation (eg, *RUNX1/AML1*, *EVI1*, or *WT1*).[45] In early-stage MDS, class I mutations are usually absent, but a variety of class II mutations may be observed.

Tumor suppressors are regulatory genes whose loss promote growth and cell cycle progression in many neoplasms. These genes can be lost by mutation, deletion, promoter methylation silencing, transcriptional regulation, or post-transcriptional mechanisms, such as microRNA targeting. Because large chromosomal deletions and chromosomal losses are common features of de novo MDS, loss of tumor suppressors by gene deletion is likely an extremely important disease mechanism in these neoplasms. To date, however, with the exception of 17p deletion that leads to the loss of *TP53* function,[46,47] tumor suppressor gene loss has not been clearly implicated in the most common MDS-associated chromosomal alterations. Instead, recent data have implicated copy number loss of genes involved in cell metabolism, such as ribosome biogenesis, protease function, and cytoskeleton regulation, in MDS pathogenesis.[46] Microarray-based gene expression profiling may help to define which gene levels are most critical and establish prognostically relevant gene signatures that correlate with French America British (FAB), WHO, or IPSS subtypes.[48,49] These studies, however, have shown considerable overlap in gene expression profiles between high-risk MDS and AML as well as between low-risk MDS and non-neoplastic conditions.

An Algorithm for Diagnosing Myelodysplastic Syndromes

Establishing a diagnosis of MDS, particularly lower-grade MDS types, in clinical cytopenia patients can be challenging. It requires that pathologists be aware of other, non-MDS causes of cytopenia and their associated changes that may mimic MDS. FCI is particularly useful in diagnostically equivocal cases. Moreover, a FCI analytic approach based mainly on CD34+ cells is highly specific for identifying stem cell neoplasms and is more straightforward for pathologists in various practice settings to interpret. When pathologists assess BM samples obtained from clinical cytopenia patients, it is recommended to follow the minimal diagnostic criteria recommended by MDS IWG and the criteria of the 2008 WHO classification. The recommended diagnostic approach for MDS is summarized in **Box 2** and a suggested diagnostic aligorithm is shown in **Fig. 5**.

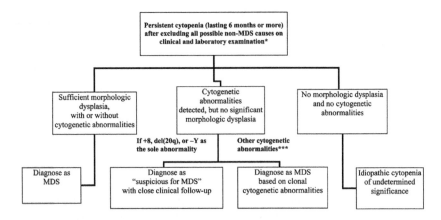

* A diagnosis of MDS can be made if cytopenia lasts <6 months but other MDS criteria are met.
** Flow cytometry immunophenotyping is particularly helpful in these cases: if abnormal results, favors MDS; if normal results, favors a benign process of cytopenia.
*** Clonal cytogenetic abnormalities, including -7, -5, del(7q), del(5q), del(11q), i(17q), -13, del(13q), del(11q), del(12p), del(9q), t(6;9)(p23;q34), and/or any translocation involving 3q, 11q, 12p, or 17p.

Fig. 5. Diagnostic algorithm for evaluating cytopenia patients to establish or exclude a diagnosis of MDS.

For many patients, diagnosing MDS using the 2008 WHO criteria is straightforward. Diagnosis can be challenging, however, when (1) there is no detectable cytogenetic abnormality and only mild cytopenia; (2) there are both a karyotypic abnormality and cytopenia but only minimal morphologic dysplasia; or (3) there is isolated persistent thrombocytopenia, neutropenia, or transfusion-dependent macrocytic anemia but no karyotypic abnormality or overt morphologic dysplasia. Therefore, an international working conference composed of representatives from the National Comprehensive Cancer Network, the International MDS Working Group, and the European LeukemiaNet proposed consensus guidelines for the minimal diagnostic criteria for MDS (see **Box 2**). A MDS diagnosis can be established when both prerequisite criteria and at least one decisive criterion are fulfilled. If no decisive criterion is fulfilled, the co-criteria should be applied. Some patients may have MDS coexisting with another hematologic or nonhematologic disease; therefore, detection of another disease potentially causing cytopenia does not exclude a diagnosis of MDS.

Patients presenting with persistent cytopenia (lasting 6 months or more) that cannot be explained by any other disease but lacking the full diagnostic criteria for MDS may be classified as idiopathic cytopenia of undetermined significance (ICUS), a newly coined term.[15,50] ICUS is a diagnosis of exclusion requiring careful BM examination, chromosome analysis and a thorough search of underlying causes. Careful follow-up is advised: approximately 20% to 50% of patients with ICUS eventually progress to MDS or AML.[50,51] FCI may be helpful in distinguishing a stem cell neoplasm versus reactive cytopenia in such cases.[30] A recent study has showed that stem cell clonality is detected in a significant subset of ICUS patients by human androgen receptor gene-based assay.[51]

In patients with persistent cytopenia, BM may show a clonal karyotypic abnormality but minimal (less than 10%) morphologic dysplasia. The 2008 WHO classification suggests handling these cases based on the type of cytogenetic change seen. When the sole aberration is −Y, +8, or del(20q), the recommendation is to diagnose these cases as suspicious for MDS, because such changes can occasionally be encountered in metaphases analysis of non-neoplastic BM, such as aplastic anemia

(AA) or idiopathic thrombocytopenic purpura (ITP).[52] The finding of any other cytogenetic abnormality is regarded as presumptive evidence for MDS.

DIFFERENTIAL DIAGNOSIS
Non-MDS Causes of Cytopenia

Common reactive causes of cytopenia are often diagnosed clinically by hematologists through a detailed history, physical examination, and laboratory tests to exclude iron, vitamin B_{12}, and folate deficiencies as well as possible effects of a drug, known infection, well-characterized autoimmune disease, hemolytic anemia, or splenomegaly. Most such patients do not require a BM biopsy. However, when cytopenia is chronic, refractory to treatment, or if clinical work-up is unrevealing, hematologists often perform a BM biopsy to rule out MDS or a BM infiltrative process.[3,4] A listing of the many non-MDS causes of various cytopenias is provided in **Table 2**.

Isolated anemia is most common and can be attributed to nutritional deficiency, systemic diseases (infections, chronic liver disease, kidney disease, collagen vascular diseases, or tumor paraneoplastic syndromes), peripheral destruction/consumption (hemolysis, splenomegaly, or microangiopathy), undiagnosed hemoglobinopathy, AA, or paroxysmal nocturnal hemoglobinuria (PNH). MDS should be a diagnosis of exclusion in these cases.

Isolated thrombocytopenia is mostly due to ITP. In children, most cases of ITP are acute, manifesting a few weeks after a viral illness. In adults, most cases of ITP are chronic, manifesting with an insidious onset, and typically occur in middle-aged women. In these patients, ITP is mediated by autoantibodies that are directed against platelet GPIIb/IIIa or GPIb/IX GP complexes (in 75% of cases).[53] Isolated thrombocytopenia is less commonly a presenting manifestation of MDS, acute leukemia, or BM failure syndromes.[54] Isolated thrombocytopenia with minimal morphologic dysplasia may occur in indolent forms of MDS, particularly in patients with a del(20q)[7] cytogenetic abnormality.

Isolated neutropenia is an uncommon presentation of MDS. The most common causes of isolated neutropenia are chemical exposure, infections, autoimmune diseases, side effect of drugs, lymphoid neoplasms, and thyroid disease.[55] The drugs associated with isolated neutropenia include the antipsychotic medication clozapine; immunosuppressive drugs, such as sirolimus, mycophenolate mofetil, tacrolimus, and cyclosporine; interferons used to treat multiple sclerosis and hepatitis C; antidepressant drugs; antibiotics; antiepilepsy drugs; and arsenic. Autoimmune neutropenia can be either primary or secondary: primary autoimmune neutropenia is often seen in children, whereas secondary autoimmune leukopenia is usually seen in adults and is associated with systemic autoimmune diseases, infections, or malignancies. Antineutrophil autoantibodies may not be detectable, because the sensitivity for antibody detection varies depending on the tests, and in some patients, autoantibodies disappear even before the patient recovers. Cyclic neutropenia is an autosomal dominant disorder of unknown etiology in which 3 to 6 days of neutropenia occur every 21 to 30 days in a periodic pattern. Of the lymphoid neoplasms, large granular lymphocytic (LGL) leukemia often presents as an isolated neutropenia.

Chronic bicytopenia and pancytopenia are more clinically suggesting of MDS, but the most common causes are still of secondary (nonhematopoietic stem cell) origin, such as infection, chronic systemic diseases, toxins or drugs, nutritional deficiencies, or hemophagocytic syndromes. In patients who have received chemotherapy for primary malignancies, complete blood counts often recover within 3 to 4 weeks. Prolonged myelosuppression may occur in some patients, however. The severity and duration of anemia, thrombocytopenia, and neutropenia differ with each patient and

Table 2
Causes of clinical cytopenia not attributed to myelodysplastic syndromes

Isolated Anemia	Isolated Thrombocytopenia	Isolated Neutropenia	Bicytopenia and Pancytopenia
Iron deficiency (including blood loss)	Idiopathic thrombocytopenia purpura	Post infectious	Post infectious
Vitamin B$_{12}$ and folate deficiency	Post infectious	Drug-induced	Drug-induced
Anemia of systemic diseases	Drug/toxin Chemotherapy/ radiation	Primary immune disorders	Nutritional deficiency
Infections	Alcohol	Antineutrophil antibodies	Aplastic anemia
Drug/toxin	Hypersplenism	Transfusion alloantibodies	Paroxysmal nocturnal hemoglobinuria
Hypersplenism	Congenital/inherited BM disorders	Antibodies to G-CSF	Macrophage activation syndrome
Hemolysis	LGL leukemia	Complement activation	Hemaphagocytosis
Aplastic anemia		Hypersplenism	Hypersplenism
Paroxysmal nocturnal hemoglobinuria		Congenital neutropenia	LGL leukemia
Low hormone:		Cyclic neutropenia	BM infiltrate:
Erythropoietin (chronic renal failure)		LGL leukemia	Hairy cell leukemia
Thyroid hormone			Other hematological/non-hematological malignancy
Androgens (hypogonadism)			Granulomas
Undiagnosed hemoglobinopathy			
Pure red cell aplasia (often due to thymoma)			
Congenital/inherited BM disorders			
Large granular lymphocytic (LGL) leukemia			

with each chemotherapy regimen and its schedule, intensity, and duration.[56] In addition, cytopenia may be attributed directly or indirectly to the primary malignancy, as a result of blood loss, paraneoplastic syndromes, malnutrition/malabsorption, altered metabolism, autoimmune phenomena, microangiopathic hemolysis,[57] secondary infection, anemia of chronic inflammation, or other causes.

Role of Bone Marrow Evaluation in Differential Diagnosis

Cytopenia due to a BM infiltrative process, such as metastatic carcinoma, lymphoma, multiple myeloma, or acute leukemia, is usually relatively straightforward for pathologists to diagnose when incorporating information from FCI and IHC. Hairy cell leukemia and LGL leukemia can be diagnostically challenging, because interstitial infiltration patterns may be subtle in the early stages of these diseases. On FCI, hairy cells in the BM samples may be underrepresented due to a poor or dry aspirate. On FCI, LGL leukemia exhibits increased numbers of LGLs, but they often have a normal immunophenotype. If there is suspicion of hairy cell leukemia or LGL leukemia, IHC for CD20, DBA-44, and annexin A1 (hairy cell leukemia) and/or for CD4, CD8, granzyme, TIA-1, and CD57 (LGL leukemia) can be helpful. BM infiltration by lymphomas can elicit a sympathetic morphologic dysplasia in the hematopoietic elements and may lead to misdiagnosis of MDS.[58,59] Most reactive morphologic dysplasia is limited to the erythroid lineage, although mild dysplasia in granulocytes and megakaryocytes can also be observed.

Cytopenia due to peripheral destruction or consumption often shows a hyperplastic and/or regenerative BM. In a briskly regenerating BM, dysplastic features may be observed. In patients with hemolytic anemia, dyserythropoiesis (so-called stress erythropoiesis) is a common feature. Dysplastic features in myeloid and megakaryocytic cells may be present in regenerating BM after chemotherapy or other marrow insults, but the changes are usually mild. In patients with drug/toxin- or autoimmune-related neutropenia, however, the myeloid series is often left-shifted and may demonstrate hypogranulation or contain abnormally coarse granules (**Fig. 6**). FCI can be particularly helpful in these cases. In patients with ITP, many young megakaryocytes are often present that are monolobated but hypergranular; these megakaryocytes should not be confused with dysplastic megakaryocytes that are both monolobated and hypogranular. Unlike MDS, which usually exhibits architectural disorganization of hemopoiesis, reactive BM samples typically maintain a relatively normal BM topography, with intact clusters of erythroid elements and megakaryocytes located away from the bone trabeculae and not forming clusters. In BM of cytopenia due to peripheral destruction,

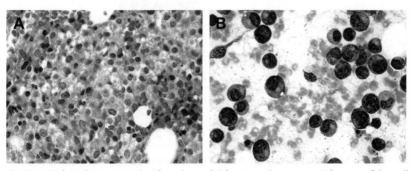

Fig. 6. Drug-induced neutropenia. There is myeloid maturation arrest with most of the cells in the promyelocyte, myelocyte, and metamyelocytes stages, seen in both the biopsy (*A*) and aspirate smear (*B*). Maturation arrest can share many clinical and morphologic features with MDS.

cytopenia correlates with specific lineage hyperplasia. For example, anemia is associated with erythroid hyperplasia, and thrombocytopenia is usually associated with megakaryocytic hyperplasia. It is important to document the number or proportion of each lineage as supporting evidence of cytopenia secondary to peripheral destruction. Reactive BM often contains increased hematogones and shows no abnormalities in CD34+ cells (see the previous FCI description), whereas MDS shows decreased or absent hematogones with aberrant expression of certain markers on myeloblasts.[60] In most cases, regenerating BM can be differentiated from MDS on a careful BM examination and a thorough review of the laboratory data.

Cytopenia due to BM suppression is more diagnostically challenging. Similar to MDS, BM samples can show increased histiocytes, apoptotic cells, and an altered stroma. These changes are particularly apparent in the BM of patients with HIV, hepatitis C virus, or systemic lupus erythematosus (**Fig. 7**) or in those who have undergone chemotherapy for malignancies. Dyserythropoiesis is commonly observed but is often mild. Dysgranulopoiesis and dysmegakaryopoiesis, if present, are also usually mild. Iron staining is helpful for identifying RS; however, storage iron is often increased in both MDS and anemia of chronic inflammation. Erythroid hypoplasia or aplasia may be indicative of a viral infection (parvovirus B19) or thymoma, but this does not exclude MDS, because erythroid hypoplasia or aplasia can be present in a subset of patients with MDS and is often associated with a clonal T-cell expansion (see **Fig. 2**C, D).[25] A cytogenetic abnormality characteristic of MDS confirms an MDS diagnosis, but cytogenetic abnormalities are only seen in 5% to 20% of patients with low-grade MDS[5] and are especially infrequent in those with RCUD (2% to 5% of cases). Alternatively, after chemotherapy and autologous stem cell transplantation, transient chromosomal abnormalities can be observed and do not predict development of t-MDS.[61,62] Therefore, these findings must be interpreted with caution. On FCI, maturing myelomonocytic cells in reactive and suppressed BM may show alterations, such as a left-shifted maturation pattern; altered CD33, CD10, CD11b, CD16, CD15, or HLA-DR expression; and/or increased CD56 expression. The CD34+ precursors are immunophenotypically normal, however, and hematogones are preserved. Nevertheless, unless the diagnosis of MDS is clear-cut, it is prudent to raise the possibility of MDS without rendering a definitive diagnosis, especially in patients who have undergone chemotherapy or stem cell transplantation. Clinical follow-up often eventually confirms a diagnosis of true MDS by establishing the chronicity of the abnormality and by allowing time for excluding other possible reactive/reversible causes.

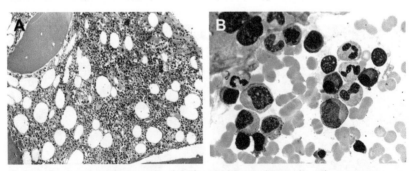

Fig. 7. Systemic lupus erythematosus. (*A*) The BM biopsy shows altered marrow stroma and some dysplastic-appearing small megakaryocytes, mimicking MDS. (*B*) Dyserythropoiesis with karyorrhexis of erythroid precursors is also present in the aspirate smear; plasma cells are increased, a clue to the diagnosis of an autoimmune disease.

Cytopenias treated with growth factors can be problematic if the growth factors are administrated empirically before a BM biopsy is conducted. The effect of growth factors complicates a BM evaluation. Granulocyte colony-stimulating factor (G-CSF) and its derivatives are widely used to reduce the duration of neutropenia induced by chemotherapy. The changes associated with G-CSF include left-shifted myeloid maturation with increased myeloid precursors, including ALIPs in some cases as a result of rapid myeloid regeneration. Cytoplasmic hypergranulation and circulating myeloid precursors and blasts can also be observed. In MDS or AML BM samples, myeloblasts can increase significantly on G-CSF stimulation and drop back to baseline after G-CSF is stopped. Thus, it is important not to overdiagnose RAEB or AML in patients who recently started G-CSF treatment. G-CSF administration causes alteration of some of flow cytometric markers, such as increased CD64 and CD14 expression and decreased CD16 expression on neutrophils, decreased side scatter of maturing myeloid cells,[63] and increased CD7+ myeloid precursors. Erythropoietin is often administrated to anemia patients with a low erythropoietin level or patients with MDS who do not have significantly increased endogenous erythropoietin levels. In reactive BM, erythropoietin often increases the proportion of erythroid cells but does not cause significant morphologic dysplasia. In contrast, erythropoietin treatment in MDS patients often leads to a decreased, rather than an increased, proportion of erythroid cells as a result of reducing apoptosis and promoting effective hematopoiesis.[64]

AA may be difficult to distinguish from hypoplastic MDS. The low cellularity **(Fig. 8**A, B) and often poor-quality aspirates obtained from such specimens make

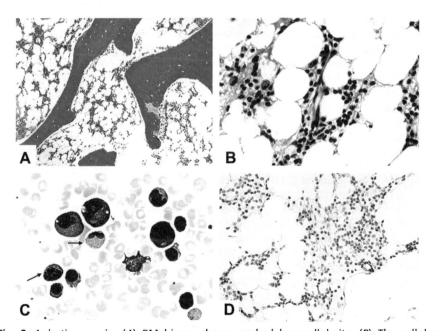

Fig. 8. Aplastic anemia. (*A*) BM biopsy shows marked hypocellularity. (*B*) The cellular elements are predominantly lymphocytes, plasma cells, stromal cells and some maturing erythroid precursors. Aplastic anemia. (*C*) Some dysplastic features can be seen in the bone marrow aspirate (*arrows*). (*D*) CD34 precursors are decreased on a CD34 immunohistochemical stain, in contrast to hypocellular MDS, in which CD34+ cells would be relatively increased.

Differential Diagnosis Myelodysplastic Syndromes	
MDS Versus	**Helpful Distinguishing Features**
Hairy cell leukemia	• CD20 immunostain reveals neoplastic B-cells in BM biopsy in an interstitial pattern
Peripheral destruction (hemolytic anemia or immune thrombocytopenia)	• Retained normal BM topography • Hyperplasia of cytopenic lineage • Normal or increased hematogones
BM suppression (infection, autoimmune disease, status post chemotherapy)	• Absence of cytogenetic abnormalities • Normal immunophenotype of CD34+ blasts • Normal or increased hematogones • Clinical history
Growth factor therapy	• Clinical history • Hypergranulation of neutrophils • Minimal or no true morphologic dysplasia
Aplastic anemia	• No increase of CD34+ cells by IHC of BM biopsy dysplasia often mild and confined to erythroid
Congenital marrow failure syndromes	• Clinical history • Absence of clonal cytogenetic abnormality • Significant morphologic dysplasia usually absent

the identification of dyspoiesis and the enumeration of blasts challenging; in some cases, it may be impossible to distinguish hypocellular MDS from AA.[65] In blood smears, macrocytic red blood cells are often found in both conditions, but the presence of neutrophils with pseudo-Pelger-Huët nuclei and/or hypogranular cytoplasm favor a diagnosis of MDS. Similarly, in BM samples, dysplastic granulopoiesis and megakaryopoiesis favor an MDS diagnosis, whereas dyserythropoiesis is less specific and can occur in AA (see **Fig. 8**C). In hypoplastic MDS, BM biopsy samples have sparsely scattered dysgranulopoietic cells, patchy islands of immature erythropoiesis, and, in most cases, decreased megakaryopoiesis with some micromegakaryocytes.[66] The BM can be completely acellular in some areas, whereas discernible dysplastic cellular islands are present in other areas. A larger and deeper biopsy may help establish a more definitive diagnosis in equivocal cases. Normal or increased CD34+ cells in the BM are more likely seen in MDS, whereas CD34+ cells are markedly decreased in AA (see **Fig. 8**D). Although the identification of a clonal chromosomal abnormality at the time of presentation is generally considered indicative of MDS, clonal chromosomal abnormalities may occasionally be seen in AA,[67] particularly in cases associated with Fanconi anemia (discussed further in Pediatric Bone Marrow Interpretation by Dr Mihaela Onciu elsewhere in this issue).[68]

Biologically, an overlap between acquired AA and hypoplastic MDS has been suggested.[69] Moreover, MDS develops in 10% to 15% of patients with AA who are not treated with hematopoietic stem cell transplantation. Small populations of clones deficient in glycophosphatidylinositol (GPI)-anchored proteins on their cell surface may be detected in 40% to 50% of patients with AA by flow cytometric analysis in the absence of clinical signs of PNH.[70] These GPI-mutated cells likely reflect an independent clonal expansion that arises because of a selective growth advantage under immune-mediated destruction of BM hematopoietic cells. However, such small clones have been detected in approximately 20% of adults with low-grade MDS.[71,72] Therefore, the presence of such a PNH cell population does not exclude a diagnosis of MDS.

Dysplastic features in inherited BM failure syndromes may mimic MDS, particularly in pediatric patients. Congenital dyserythropoietic anemia, Noonan syndrome,

Dobowitz syndrome, mitochondrial disorders (Pearson syndrome),[73] reticular dysgenesis, thrombocytopenia with absent radii syndrome, and congenital amegakaryocytic thrombocytopenia[14] can share some morphologic and clinical features with MDS but are not necessarily associated with an increased risk of acute leukemia. Many inherited BM failure disorders cannot be separated from MDS by morphologic criteria and, to make this distinction, careful physical examination, past medical history and family history analysis, and other appropriate laboratory tests are required. An associated constitutional abnormality is present in 29% to 45% of all pediatric MDS patients.[74] In patients with congenital BM failure disorders, hematopoiesis can show dysplastic features, in particular dyserythropoiesis. Therefore, evolution of MDS in such a setting can only be diagnosed if a persistent clonal chromosomal abnormality is present or if hypercellularity in the BM develops in the presence of persistent unexplained peripheral cytopenia. Diagnosis of MDS in pediatric patients is discussed in more detail in Pediatric Bone Marrow Interpretation by Dr Mihaela Onciu elsewhere, in this issue.

PROGNOSIS

The most significant causes of mortality in patients with MDS are BM failure and transformation to acute leukemia, which is almost always AML with rare cases of B lymphoblastic leukemia reported.[75,76] The overall incidence of transformation to AML in MDS is approximately 30% but varies significantly by subtype—5% to 35% for patients with RAEB compared with only 2% for refractory anemia.[77] The IPSS 4-tier score combining the percentage of marrow blasts, specific cytogenetic abnormalities, and number of cytopenias effectively predicts overall survival and evolution to AML. The median survival of patients in the IPSS-high group is only 0.4 years versus 5.7 years for patients in the IPSS-low group.[14] Several other clinical and pathologic factors have been shown to add significant prognostic information to that provided by the IPSS, such as patient age, performance status, transfusion dependence, WHO disease subtype, presence of marrow fibrosis, clustering of CD34+ myeloblasts, presence of ALIPs, and presence of molecular alterations involving *FLT3, KIT, TP53,* and *RAS* genes.[77–81] Although the presence of 20% blasts in PB or BM distinguishes AML from high-grade MDS (RAEB) according to the 2008 WHO Classification of MDS in adults, patients with lower blast counts may still be treated as AML, especially in the pediatric population. Therapeutic algorithms are currently based on a complex matrix of patient age, performance status, and risk and benefit assessment.

Pitfalls in Myelodysplastic Syndromes

! Establishing an initial diagnosis of low-grade MDS can be challenging, because cytogenetic alterations are infrequent and non-MDS cytopenias can mimic MDS morphologically.

! Because lymphomas and plasma cell myeloma may share a similar cytopenic presentation with MDS, flow cytometry panels used to evaluate cytopenic patients should include markers capable of detecting clonal B cells, aberrant T cells, and clonal plasma cells.

! The presence of a cytogenetic abnormality is not necessarily indicative of MDS.

! Patients with idiopathic cytopenia of undetermined significance (ICUS) need close clinical follow-up.

! Aplastic anemia, especially after therapy, can share many features with hypoplastic MDS.

REFERENCES

1. Adams PF, Hendershot GE, Marano MA. Current estimates from the National Health Interview Survey, 1996. Vital Health Stat 10 1999;200:1–203.
2. DeMaeyer E, Adiels-Tegman M. The prevalence of anaemia in the world. World Health Stat Q 1985;38:302–16.
3. Dubois RW, Goodnough LT, Ershler WB, et al. Identification, diagnosis, and management of anemia in adult ambulatory patients treated by primary care physicians: evidence-based and consensus recommendations. Curr Med Res Opin 2006;22:385–95.
4. Goldstein KH, Abramson N. Efficient diagnosis of thrombocytopenia. Am Fam Physician 1996;53:915–20.
5. Swerdlow SH, Campo E, Harris NL, et al, editors. WHO classification of tumours of haematopoietic and lymphoid tissues. 4th edition. Lyon (France): IARC press; 2008. p. 87.
6. Vardiman JW, Harris NL, Brunning RD. The World Health Organization (WHO) classification of the myeloid neoplasms. Blood 2002;100:2292–302.
7. Gupta R, Soupir CP, Johari V, et al. Myelodysplastic syndrome with isolated deletion of chromosome 20q: an indolent disease with minimal morphological dysplasia and frequent thrombocytopenic presentation. Br J Haematol 2007;139:265–8.
8. Kuroda J, Kimura S, Kobayashi Y, et al. Unusual myelodysplastic syndrome with the initial presentation mimicking idiopathic thrombocytopenic purpura. Acta Haematol 2002;108:139–43.
9. Vardiman JW. Hematopathological concepts and controversies in the diagnosis and classification of myelodysplastic syndromes. Hematology Am Soc Hematol Educ Program 2006;199–204.
10. Schmitt-Graeff A, Mattern D, Kohler H, et al. [Myelodysplastic syndromes (MDS). Aspects of hematopathologic diagnosis]. Pathologe 2000;21:1–15 [in German].
11. Sole F, Espinet B, Sanz GF, et al. Incidence, characterization and prognostic significance of chromosomal abnormalities in 640 patients with primary myelodysplastic syndromes. Grupo Cooperativo Espanol de Citogenetica Hematologica. Br J Haematol 2000;108:346–56.
12. Young NS, Calado RT, Scheinberg P. Current concepts in the pathophysiology and treatment of aplastic anemia. Blood 2006;108:2509–19.
13. Konoplev S, Medeiros LJ, Lennon PA, et al. Therapy may unmask hypoplastic myelodysplastic syndrome that mimics aplastic anemia. Cancer 2007;110:1520–6.
14. Greenberg P, Cox C, LeBeau MM, et al. International scoring system for evaluating prognosis in myelodysplastic syndromes. Blood 1997;89:2079–88.
15. Valent P, Horny HP, Bennett JM, et al. Definitions and standards in the diagnosis and treatment of the myelodysplastic syndromes: consensus statements and report from a working conference. Leuk Res 2007;31:727–36.
16. Verburgh E, Achten R, Louw VJ, et al. A new disease categorization of low-grade myelodysplastic syndromes based on the expression of cytopenia and dysplasia in one versus more than one lineage improves on the WHO classification. Leukemia 2007;21:668–77.
17. Verburgh E, Achten R, Maes B, et al. Additional prognostic value of bone marrow histology in patients subclassified according to the International Prognostic Scoring System for myelodysplastic syndromes. J Clin Oncol 2003;21:273–82.
18. Mangi MH, Mufti GJ. Primary myelodysplastic syndromes: diagnostic and prognostic significance of immunohistochemical assessment of bone marrow biopsies. Blood 1992;79:198–205.

19. Mangi MH, Salisbury JR, Mufti GJ. Abnormal localization of immature precursors (ALIP) in the bone marrow of myelodysplastic syndromes: current state of knowledge and future directions. Leuk Res 1991;15:627–39.
20. Ogata K, Nakamura K, Yokose N, et al. Clinical significance of phenotypic features of blasts in patients with myelodysplastic syndrome. Blood 2002;100:3887–96.
21. Oriani A, Annaloro C, Soligo D, et al. Bone marrow histology and CD34 immunostaining in the prognostic evaluation of primary myelodysplastic syndromes. Br J Haematol 1996;92:360–4.
22. Mufti GJ, Bennett JM, Goasguen J, et al. Diagnosis and classification of myelodysplastic syndrome: International Working Group on Morphology of myelodysplastic syndrome (IWGM-MDS) consensus proposals for the definition and enumeration of myeloblasts and ring sideroblasts. Haematologica 2008;93:1712–7.
23. Hasserjian RP, Zuo Z, Garcia C, et al. Acute erythroid leukemia: a reassessment using criteria refined in the 2008 WHO classification. Blood 2010;115(10): 1985–92.
24. Wang SA, Tang G, Fadare O, et al. Erythroid-predominant myelodysplastic syndromes: enumeration of blasts from nonerythroid rather than total marrow cells provides superior risk stratification. Mod Pathol 2008;21:1394–402.
25. Wang SA, Yue G, Hutchinson L, et al. Myelodysplastic syndrome with pure red cell aplasia shows characteristic clinicopathological features and clonal T-cell expansion. Br J Haematol 2007;138:271–5.
26. Shimamoto T, Iguchi T, Ando K, et al. Successful treatment with cyclosporin A for myelodysplastic syndrome with erythroid hypoplasia associated with T-cell receptor gene rearrangements. Br J Haematol 2001;114:358–61.
27. Kussick SJ, Fromm JR, Rossini A, et al. Four-color flow cytometry shows strong concordance with bone marrow morphology and cytogenetics in the evaluation for myelodysplasia. Am J Clin Pathol 2005;124:170–81.
28. Stachurski D, Smith BR, Pozdnyakova O, et al. Flow cytometric analysis of myelomonocytic cells by a pattern recognition approach is sensitive and specific in diagnosing myelodysplastic syndrome and related marrow diseases: emphasis on a global evaluation and recognition of diagnostic pitfalls. Leuk Res 2008;32:215–24.
29. Wells DA, Benesch M, Loken MR, et al. Myeloid and monocytic dyspoiesis as determined by flow cytometric scoring in myelodysplastic syndrome correlates with the IPSS and with outcome after hematopoietic stem cell transplantation. Blood 2003;102:394–403.
30. Truong F, Smith BR, Stachurski D, et al. The utility of flow cytometric immunophenotyping in cytopenic patients with a non-diagnostic bone marrow: a prospective study. Leuk Res 2009;33:1039–46.
31. Ogata K, Della Porta MG, Malcovati L, et al. Diagnostic utility of flow cytometry in low-grade myelodysplastic syndromes: a prospective validation study. Haematologica 2009;94:1066–74.
32. van de Loosdrecht AA, Alhan C, Bene MC, et al. Standardization of flow cytometry in myelodysplastic syndromes: report from the first European LeukemiaNet working conference on flow cytometry in myelodysplastic syndromes. Haematologica 2009;94:1124–34.
33. Ogata K, Kishikawa Y, Satoh C, et al. Diagnostic application of flow cytometric characteristics of CD34+ cells in low-grade myelodysplastic syndromes. Blood 2006;108:1037–44.
34. Haase D, Germing U, Schanz J, et al. New insights into the prognostic impact of the karyotype in MDS and correlation with subtypes: evidence from a core dataset of 2124 patients. Blood 2007;110:4385–95.

35. Pozdnyakova O, Miron PM, Tang G, et al. Cytogenetic abnormalities in a series of 1,029 patients with primary myelodysplastic syndromes: a report from the US with a focus on some undefined single chromosomal abnormalities. Cancer 2008;113: 3331–40.

36. Sole F, Luno E, Sanzo C, et al. Identification of novel cytogenetic markers with prognostic significance in a series of 968 patients with primary myelodysplastic syndromes. Haematologica 2005;90:1168–78.

37. Haase D. Cytogenetic features in myelodysplastic syndromes. Ann Hematol 2008;87:515–26.

38. Beyer V, Castagne C, Muhlematter D, et al. Systematic screening at diagnosis of -5/del(5)(q31), -7, or chromosome 8 aneuploidy by interphase fluorescence in situ hybridization in 110 acute myelocytic leukemia and high-risk myelodysplastic syndrome patients: concordances and discrepancies with conventional cytogenetics. Cancer Genet Cytogenet 2004;152:29–41.

39. Yang W, Stotler B, Sevilla DW, et al. FISH analysis in addition to G-band karyotyping: Utility in evaluation of myelodysplastic syndromes? Leuk Res 2010;34(4):420–5.

40. Cuneo A, Bigoni R, Roberti MG, et al. Detection and monitoring of trisomy 8 by fluorescence in situ hybridization in acute myeloid leukemia: a multicentric study. Haematologica 1998;83:21–6.

41. Paulsson K, Heidenblad M, Strombeck B, et al. High-resolution genome-wide array-based comparative genome hybridization reveals cryptic chromosome changes in AML and MDS cases with trisomy 8 as the sole cytogenetic aberration. Leukemia 2006;20:840–6.

42. Evers C, Beier M, Poelitz A, et al. Molecular definition of chromosome arm 5q deletion end points and detection of hidden aberrations in patients with myelodysplastic syndromes and isolated del(5q) using oligonucleotide array CGH. Genes Chromosomes Cancer 2007;46:1119–28.

43. Maciejewski JP, Mufti GJ. Whole genome scanning as a cytogenetic tool in hematologic malignancies. Blood 2008;112:965–74.

44. Makishima H, Rataul M, Gondek LP, et al. FISH and SNP-A karyotyping in myelodysplastic syndromes: improving cytogenetic detection of del(5q), monosomy 7, del(7q), trisomy 8 and del(20q). Leuk Res 2010;34(4):447–53.

45. Deguchi K, Gilliland DG. Cooperativity between mutations in tyrosine kinases and in hematopoietic transcription factors in AML. Leukemia 2002;16:740–4.

46. Bernasconi P. Molecular pathways in myelodysplastic syndromes and acute myeloid leukemia: relationships and distinctions-a review. Br J Haematol 2008;142:695–708.

47. Sankar M, Tanaka K, Kumaravel TS, et al. Identification of a commonly deleted region at 17p13.3 in leukemia and lymphoma associated with 17 p abnormality. Leukemia 1998;12:510–6.

48. Pellagatti A, Esoof N, Watkins F, et al. Gene expression profiling in the myelodysplastic syndromes using cDNA microarray technology. Br J Haematol 2004;125: 576–83.

49. Hofmann WK, de Vos S, Komor M, et al. Characterization of gene expression of CD34+ cells from normal and myelodysplastic bone marrow. Blood 2002;100: 3553–60.

50. Wimazal F, Fonatsch C, Thalhammer R, et al. Idiopathic cytopenia of undetermined significance (ICUS) versus low risk MDS: the diagnostic interface. Leuk Res 2007;31:1461–8.

51. Schroeder T, Ruf L, Bernhardt A, et al. Distinguishing myelodysplastic syndromes (MDS) from idiopathic cytopenia of undetermined significance (ICUS): HUMARA unravels clonality in a subgroup of patients. Ann Oncol 2010;21(11):2267–71.

52. Soupir CP, Vergilio JA, Kelly E, et al. Identification of del(20q) in a subset of patients diagnosed with idiopathic thrombocytopenic purpura. Br J Haematol 2009;144:800–2.
53. Tani P, Berchtold P, McMillan R. Autoantibodies in chronic ITP. Blut 1989;59:44–6.
54. Sashida G, Takaku TI, Shoji N, et al. Clinico-hematologic features of myelodysplastic syndrome presenting as isolated thrombocytopenia: an entity with a relatively favorable prognosis. Leuk Lymphoma 2003;44:653–8.
55. Lima CS, Paula EV, Takahashi T, et al. Causes of incidental neutropenia in adulthood. Ann Hematol 2006;85:705–9.
56. Daniel D, Crawford J. Myelotoxicity from chemotherapy. Semin Oncol 2006;33: 74–85.
57. Lin YC, Chang HK, Sun CF, et al. Microangiopathic hemolytic anemia as an initial presentation of metastatic cancer of unknown primary origin. Southampt Med J 1995;88:683–7.
58. Pittaluga S, Verhoef G, Maes A, et al. Bone marrow trephines. Findings in patients with hairy cell leukaemia before and after treatment. Histopathology 1994;25: 129–35.
59. Castello A, Coci A, Magrini U. Paraneoplastic marrow alterations in patients with cancer. Haematologica 1992;77:392–7.
60. Maftoun-Banankhah S, Maleki A, Karandikar NJ, et al. Multiparameter flow cytometric analysis reveals low percentage of bone marrow hematogones in myelodysplastic syndromes. Am J Clin Pathol 2008;129:300–8.
61. Martinez-Climent JA, Comes AM, Vizcarra E, et al. Chromosomal abnormalities in women with breast cancer after autologous stem cell transplantation are infrequent and may not predict development of therapy-related leukemia or myelodysplastic syndrome. Bone Marrow Transplant 2000;25:1203–8.
62. Imrie KR, Dube I, Prince HM, et al. New clonal karyotypic abnormalities acquired following autologous bone marrow transplantation for acute myeloid leukemia do not appear to confer an adverse prognosis. Bone Marrow Transplant 1998;21:395–9.
63. Carulli G. Effects of recombinant human granulocyte colony-stimulating factor administration on neutrophil phenotype and functions. Haematologica 1997;82: 606–16.
64. Hellstrom-Lindberg E, Kanter-Lewensohn L, Ost A. Morphological changes and apoptosis in bone marrow from patients with myelodysplastic syndromes treated with granulocyte-CSF and erythropoietin. Leuk Res 1997;21:415–25.
65. Hasle H, Baumann I, Bergstrasser E, et al. The International Prognostic Scoring System (IPSS) for childhood myelodysplastic syndrome (MDS) and juvenile myelomonocytic leukemia (JMML). Leukemia 2004;18:2008–14.
66. Meadows AT, Baum E, Fossati-Bellani F, et al. Second malignant neoplasms in children: an update from the late effects Study Group. J Clin Oncol 1985;3:532–8.
67. Bhatia S, Ramsay NK, Steinbuch M, et al. Malignant neoplasms following bone marrow transplantation. Blood 1996;87:3633–9.
68. Neglia JP, Friedman DL, Yasui Y, et al. Second malignant neoplasms in five-year survivors of childhood cancer: childhood cancer survivor study. J Natl Cancer Inst 2001;93:618–29.
69. Barrett J, Saunthararajah Y, Molldrem J. Myelodysplastic syndrome and aplastic anemia: distinct entities or diseases linked by a common pathophysiology? Semin Hematol 2000;37:15–29.
70. Maciejewski JP, Rivera C, Kook H, et al. Relationship between bone marrow failure syndromes and the presence of glycophosphatidyl inositol-anchored protein-deficient clones. Br J Haematol 2001;115:1015–22.

71. Wang SA, Pozdnyakova O, Jorgensen JL, et al. Detection of paroxysmal nocturnal hemoglobinuria clones in patients with myelodysplastic syndromes and related bone marrow diseases, with emphasis on diagnostic pitfalls and caveats. Haematologica 2009;94:29–37.

72. Wang H, Chuhjo T, Yasue S, et al. Clinical significance of a minor population of paroxysmal nocturnal hemoglobinuria-type cells in bone marrow failure syndrome. Blood 2002;100:3897–902.

73. Passmore SJ, Hann IM, Stiller CA, et al. Pediatric myelodysplasia: a study of 68 children and a new prognostic scoring system. Blood 1995;85:1742–50.

74. Bacigalupo A, Broccia G, Corda G, et al. Antilymphocyte globulin, cyclosporin, and granulocyte colony-stimulating factor in patients with acquired severe aplastic anemia (SAA): a pilot study of the EBMT SAA Working Party. Blood 1995;85:1348–53.

75. Disperati P, Ichim CV, Tkachuk D, et al. Progression of myelodysplasia to acute lymphoblastic leukaemia: implications for disease biology. Leuk Res 2006;30:233–9.

76. Zainina S, Cheong SK. Myelodysplastic syndrome transformed into Acute Lymphoblastic Leukaemia (FAB: L3). Clin Lab Haematol 2006;28:282–3.

77. Malcovati L, Germing U, Kuendgen A, et al. Time-dependent prognostic scoring system for predicting survival and leukemic evolution in myelodysplastic syndromes. J Clin Oncol 2007;25:3503–10.

78. Kantarjian H, O'Brien S, Ravandi F, et al. Proposal for a new risk model in myelodysplastic syndrome that accounts for events not considered in the original International Prognostic Scoring System. Cancer 2008;113:1351–61.

79. Balducci L. Transfusion independence in patients with myelodysplastic syndromes: impact on outcomes and quality of life. Cancer 2006;106:2087–94.

80. Shih LY, Lin TL, Wang PN, et al. Internal tandem duplication of fms-like tyrosine kinase 3 is associated with poor outcome in patients with myelodysplastic syndrome. Cancer 2004;101:989–98.

81. Kita-Sasai Y, Horiike S, Misawa S, et al. International prognostic scoring system and TP53 mutations are independent prognostic indicators for patients with myelodysplastic syndrome. Br J Haematol 2001;115:309–12.

Index

Note: Page numbers of article titles are in **boldface** type.

A

Allogeneic stem cell transplantation, for CML, **1025–1048**
    role of in era of TKIs, 1028–1040
        changing paradigm, 1028–1029
        combined with imatinib as frontline therapy in chronic phase, 1029–1034
        conditioning regimen, 1035–1036
        current recommendations, 1039–1040
        management of hematologic relapse after, 1037–1038
        methods of, and patient selection for, 1034–1040
        monitoring after, 1036
        prevention of early treatment of disease recurrence with TKIs or cellular therapy
          after, 1037
        prognostic scoring system, 1034
        role of stem cell harvesting and autologous stem cell transplant, 1038–1039
        sibling *vs.* unrelated donor, 1035
        source of stem cells, 1034–1035
    role of in pre-TKI era, 1025–1028
Aspirates, bone marrow, in diagnosis of MDS in cytopenic patients, 1090–1092
Autologous stem cell transplantation, role of, in CML treatment, 1038–1039

B

BCR-ABL inhibitors, measuring sensitivity to, in selection of CML therapy, 1013
BCR-ABL mutations, as factor in selection of therapy for CML, 1009–1023
        dynamics of, 1000–1004
        incidence of, 1000
        methods of detection of, 998
        types of, 998–1000
    dynamics of, after imatinib cessation, 1002–1003
        during dasatinib and nilotinib therapy, 1003–1004
        during imatinib treatment, 1000–1002
    types of, ABL polymorphisms, 999
        deletion mutations, 999
        point mutations, 998–999
Biology, of CML progression, **967–980**
Biopsy, bone marrow, in diagnosis of MDS in cytopenic patients, 1089–1090
Blast crisis, allogeneic stem cell transplantation for patients in, 1032
    in biology of CML progression, **967–980**
Bone marrow, *versus* peripheral blood as source of stem cells for transplant in CML,
    1034–1035
Bone marrow aspirate, in diagnosis of MDS in cytopenic patients, 1090–1092

Hematol Oncol Clin N Am 25 (2011) 1111–1118
doi:10.1016/S0889-8588(11)00127-4
0889-8588/11/$ – see front matter © 2011 Elsevier Inc. All rights reserved.

hemonc.theclinics.com

United States Postal Service

Statement of Ownership, Management, and Circulation
(All Periodicals Publications Except Requestor Publications)

1. Publication Title	2. Publication Number	3. Filing Date
Hematology/Oncology Clinics of North America	0 0 2 - 4 7 3	9/16/11

4. Issue Frequency	5. Number of Issues Published Annually	6. Annual Subscription Price
Feb, Apr, Jun, Aug, Oct, Dec	6	$327.00

7. Complete Mailing Address of Known Office of Publication (Not printer) (Street, city, county, state, and ZIP+4®)

Elsevier Inc.
360 Park Avenue South
New York, NY 10010-1710

Contact Person
Stephen Bushing

Telephone (Include area code)
215-239-3688

8. Complete Mailing Address of Headquarters or General Business Office of Publisher (Not printer)

Elsevier Inc., 360 Park Avenue South, New York, NY 10010-1710

9. Full Names and Complete Mailing Addresses of Publisher, Editor, and Managing Editor (Do not leave blank)

Publisher (Name and complete mailing address)

Kim Murphy, Elsevier, Inc., 1600 John F. Kennedy Blvd. Suite 1800, Philadelphia, PA 19103-2899

Editor (Name and complete mailing address)

Patrick Manley, Elsevier, Inc., 1600 John F. Kennedy Blvd. Suite 1800, Philadelphia, PA 19103-2899

Managing Editor (Name and complete mailing address)

Barton Dudlick, Elsevier, Inc., 1600 John F. Kennedy Blvd. Suite 1800, Philadelphia, PA 19103-2899

10. Owner (Do not leave blank. If the publication is owned by a corporation, give the name and address of the corporation immediately followed by the names and addresses of all stockholders owning or holding 1 percent or more of the total amount of stock. If not owned by a corporation, give the names and addresses of the individual owners. If owned by a partnership or other unincorporated firm, give its name and address as well as those of each individual owner. If the publication is published by a nonprofit organization, give its name and address.)

Full Name	Complete Mailing Address
Wholly owned subsidiary of	4520 East-West Highway
Reed/Elsevier, US holdings	Bethesda, MD 20814

11. Known Bondholders, Mortgagees, and Other Security Holders Owning or Holding 1 Percent or More of Total Amount of Bonds, Mortgages, or Other Securities. If none, check box. ☐ None

Full Name	Complete Mailing Address
N/A	

12. Tax Status (For completion by nonprofit organizations authorized to mail at nonprofit rates) (Check one)
The purpose, function, and nonprofit status of this organization and the exempt status for federal income tax purposes:
☐ Has Not Changed During Preceding 12 Months
☐ Has Changed During Preceding 12 Months (Publisher must submit explanation of change with this statement)

PS Form 3526, September 2007 (Page 1 of 3 (Instructions Page 3)) PSN 7530-01-000-9931 PRIVACY NOTICE: See our Privacy policy in www.usps.com

13. Publication Title	14. Issue Date for Circulation Data Below
Hematology/Oncology Clinics of North America	August 2011

15. Extent and Nature of Circulation			Average No. Copies Each Issue During Preceding 12 Months	No. Copies of Single Issue Published Nearest to Filing Date
a. Total Number of Copies (Net press run)			1564	1400
b. Paid Circulation (By Mail and Outside the Mail)	(1)	Mailed Outside-County Paid Subscriptions Stated on PS Form 3541. (Include paid distribution above nominal rate, advertiser's proof copies, and exchange copies)	448	423
	(2)	Mailed In-County Paid Subscriptions Stated on PS Form 3541 (Include paid distribution above nominal rate, advertiser's proof copies, and exchange copies)		
	(3)	Paid Distribution Outside the Mails Including Sales Through Dealers and Carriers, Street Vendors, Counter Sales, and Other Paid Distribution Outside USPS®	266	295
	(4)	Paid Distribution by Other Classes Mailed Through the USPS (e.g. First-Class Mail®)		
c. Total Paid Distribution (Sum of 15b (1), (2), (3), and (4))		▶	714	718
d. Free or Nominal Rate Distribution (By Mail and Outside the Mail)	(1)	Free or Nominal Rate Outside-County Copies Included on PS Form 3541	118	113
	(2)	Free or Nominal Rate In-County Copies Included on PS Form 3541		
	(3)	Free or Nominal Rate Copies Mailed at Other Classes Through the USPS (e.g. First-Class Mail)		
	(4)	Free or Nominal Rate Distribution Outside the Mail (Carriers or other means)		
e. Total Free or Nominal Rate Distribution (Sum of 15d (1), (2), (3) and (4))		▶	118	113
f. Total Distribution (Sum of 15c and 15e)		▶	832	831
g. Copies not Distributed (See instructions to publishers #4 (page 83))		▶	732	569
h. Total (Sum of 15f and g)		▶	1564	1400
i. Percent Paid (15c divided by 15f times 100)			85.82%	86.40%

16. Publication of Statement of Ownership
☐ If the publication is a general publication, publication of this statement is required. Will be printed ☐ Publication not required
in the October 2011 issue of this publication.

17. Signature and Title of Editor, Publisher, Business Manager, or Owner	Date
[signature] Stephen R. Bushing – Inventory/Distribution Coordinator	September 16, 2011

I certify that all information furnished on this form is true and complete. I understand that anyone who furnishes false or misleading information on this form or who omits material or information requested on the form may be subject to criminal sanctions (including fines and imprisonment) and/or civil sanctions (including civil penalties).

PS Form 3526, September 2007 (Page 2 of 3)

Moving?

Make sure your subscription moves with you!

To notify us of your new address, find your **Clinics Account Number** (located on your mailing label above your name), and contact customer service at:

Email: journalscustomerservice-usa@elsevier.com

800-654-2452 (subscribers in the U.S. & Canada)
314-447-8871 (subscribers outside of the U.S. & Canada)

Fax number: 314-447-8029

Elsevier Health Sciences Division
Subscription Customer Service
3251 Riverport Lane
Maryland Heights, MO 63043

*To ensure uninterrupted delivery of your subscription, please notify us at least 4 weeks in advance of move.

Printed and bound by CPI Group (UK) Ltd, Croydon, CR0 4YY

03/10/2024

01040461-0015